Managing COPD

Third edition

Managing COPD
Third edition

Richard EK Russell
Imperial College London, UK

Paul A Ford
Imperial College London, UK

Peter J Barnes
National Heart and Lung Institute, Imperial College London, London, UK

Sarah Russell
Hospice of St Francis Berkhamsted, UK

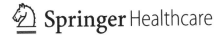

Published by Springer Healthcare Ltd, 236 Gray's Inn Road, London, WC1X 8HB, UK.

www.springerhealthcare.com

©2013 Springer Healthcare, a part of Springer Science+Business Media.

British Library Cataloguing-in-Publication Data.

A catalogue record for this book is available from the British Library.

ISBN 978-1-908517-69-2

Project editor: Tamsin Curtis
Designer: Joe Harvey
Artworker: Sissan Mollerfors
Production: Marina Maher
Printed in Singapore by Stamford Press

Contents

Author biographies

Richard EK Russell, FRCP, PhD, is Honorary Clinical Senior Lecturer at Imperial College, London, UK. He trained at Guy's Hospital and then further in Respiratory Medicine in South London and the Royal Brompton Hospitals. He has been a Consultant at Wexham Park and Windsor Hospitals for 4 years with special interests in chronic obstructive pulmonary disease (COPD), particularly its pathophysiology, asthma and delivery of care across the primary/secondary care interface. Dr Russell completed a PhD as a British Lung Foundation Research Fellow. The primary area of research was into basic mechanisms of COPD and disease progression in smokers in primary care. This is a continuing area of study for Dr Russell. He is active in the British Thoracic Society and the British Lung Foundation. Dr Russell is the lead from secondary care on the primary care quality outcomes framework national working party.

Paul A Ford, MRCP, PhD, is MRC Senior Clinical Research Fellow at Imperial College and Honorary Clinical Fellow at the Royal Brompton, and Wexham and Heatherwood NHS trusts. Dr Ford qualified from St. George's Hospital Medical School, London, in 1990 and completed his PhD in 2003 in Cellular Biology at Imperial College and Royal Brompton NHS trust. His thesis was primarily concerned with the role of the macrophage in airway inflammation, particularly COPD. Currently, he is working on developing novel pharmacological therapies for the treatment of COPD; in particular, modulating airway inflammation.

Peter J Barnes, FMedSci, FRS, is Professor of Thoracic Medicine at Imperial College London, UK. Prof. Barnes runs a large and active multidisciplinary group of over 80 researchers exploring the mechanisms and treatment of asthma and more recently COPD. He has linked molecular and cell biology to clinical studies in order to understand the inflammatory process in airway disease and to understand the mechanisms of action of currently used drugs. He has also pioneered the use of noninvasive markers to monitor lung inflammation, which has enabled research into inflammatory mechanisms to be extended to patients with severe disease. Prof. Barnes has published over 1000 papers in peer-reviewed journals and has written, edited or co-edited over 30 books on airway diseases and lung pharmacology. He serves on the editorial boards of more than 20 international journals and on several national and international advisory boards, and is a member of the scientific committees for the Global Initiative for Chronic Obstructive Lung Disease (GOLD) and Global Initiative for Asthma (GINA) guidelines.

Sarah Russell qualified as a Nurse at Guys and Lewisham NHS Trust in 1989 and has worked in the primary, secondary and palliative care charity sector as a palliative care clinical nurse specialist, team leader and multi professional educator. Sarah has a particular interest in education, communication skills, advance care planning and palliative care of Chronic Obstructive Pulmonary Disease. Sarah is currently completing a 6 year part time Doctorate in Health Research involving a narrative video research methodology regarding advance care planning entitled *'What would influence patients to discuss their preferences and wishes about care at the end of life'*.

Chapter 1

Introduction

Welcome to a revised guide for use in the management of patients with chronic obstructive pulmonary disease (COPD). We have attempted to take a fresh approach to this disease, with the aim of concentrating on the numerous effects that COPD can have on a patient.

An understanding of the pathological processes involved in the aetiology of COPD underpins effective disease management. In particular, given the disease's wide heterogeneity, a better understanding of the innate and adaptive processes underpinning the complex small airway inflammation will lead to more effective therapies. This knowledge must be applied appropriately, with 'tailored' treatment fitted to individual patients and their disease.

The history of COPD

The terms 'chronic bronchitis' and 'emphysema' were formally defined at a CIBA (Gesellschaft für Chemische Industrie Basel) guest symposium of physicians in 1959, and it is believed that the term COPD was first mentioned by William Briscoe in discussion at the 9th Aspen Emphysema Conference in 1965. This has gradually overtaken other terms to become established today as the preferred name for the disease. Nevertheless, it is important to realise that, in reality, COPD is an 'umbrella term' and describes a heterogeneous group of diseases with similar manifestations, including overlapping disease processes such as chronic bronchitis, emphysema, asthma, bronchiectasis and bronchiolitis.

Bonet, with his description of 'voluminous lungs' in 1679, is often credited with the first accurate description of emphysema, and Ruysh

R. E. K. Russell et al., *Managing COPD*,
DOI: 10.1007/978-1-907673-52-8_1, © Springer Healthcare 2013

(1721) with the first accurate illustration of enlarged air spaces. However, it is also worth bearing in mind that the Greek term *aazein* or 'sharp breath' is first described in Homer's Iliad around 2000 years earlier. The Chinese have probably used ephedrine to treat airway obstruction for just as long, and both Hippocrates (460–357 BC) and Galen (201–130 BC) established that asthma (and quite possibly COPD) is caused by bronchial obstruction. Rene Laennec, in his book *Treatise of Diseases of the Chest* (1821), described lungs that did not collapse at autopsy and theorised that this air trapping occurred because of greater inspiratory forces overcoming weaker expiratory ones. It was an eloquent concept that was subsequently disproved, as we now know that the respiratory system can develop much greater expiratory than inspiratory forces. Einthoven correctly postulated the hallmark expiratory flow resistance in COPD as early as 1892, but it was Dayman in 1951 who was the first to measure this increase in expiratory resistance, ie, give an accurate physiological explanation of dynamic expiratory airflow collapse. The more recent work of James Hogg has further advanced our understanding of the role that small airways play in the pathogenesis of the disease [1,2].

What are the goals of therapy in COPD?

Achieving defined outcomes in COPD disease management is a challenging problem. Lung function in relatively young smokers can improve significantly after smoking cessation, but restoring lung function back to normal is not usually an option. Stepwise treatment algorithms exist for COPD as they do for asthma, but smoking cessation is the only proven effective disease-modifying intervention (Figure 1.1) [3]. However, smoking is not the only causal mechanism; the World Health Organisation (WHO) estimates that nearly 25% of global COPD burden is caused by the use of indoor biomass fuels in developing countries.

Unlike treatment for asthma, treatment for COPD is often without immediate clinical benefit and can seem relatively unrewarding for practitioners. Thus, therapy goals should be realistic. We now understand that evaluating the effects of new therapies in COPD can take many months, and more emphasis may be placed on outcome measures such as quality of life (QOL) and exacerbation rates/severity than more traditional

Effects of sustained smoking cessation on FEV$_1$

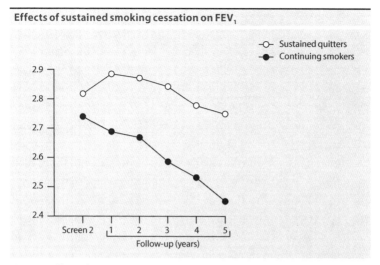

Figure 1.1 Effects of sustained smoking cessation on FEV$_1$. Mean post-bronchodilator forced expiratory volume at 1 s (FEV$_1$) for participants in the smoking intervention and placebo group who were sustained quitters and continuing smokers. The two curves diverge sharply after baseline. Reproduced with permission from AMA [3].

spirometric measures. Unfortunately, patients generally present late in the course of their disease, when they are often quite debilitated and less can be done to affect long-term outcome.

The Global Initiative for Chronic Obstructive Lung Disease (GOLD) has produced guidelines for the management of COPD [4]. The aims of therapy wherever possible are to:

- prevent disease progression;
- relieve symptoms;
- improve exercise tolerance;
- improve health status;
- prevent and treat exacerbations; and
- reduce mortality.

The Food and Drug Administration (FDA) has also introduced its own 'wish lists' for outcome measures in COPD, including acute exacerbations of chronic bronchitis [5,6]. By concentrating on these goals with a consistent and realistic approach, even the most disabled patients are capable of remarkable improvements in QOL.

What is achievable in primary care?

COPD is a very common condition. In any population where cigarette smoking is prevalent, COPD will be present. According to global WHO estimates, 80 million people have moderate to severe COPD and in 2005 3 million people died of COPD. The WHO predicts that COPD will become the third leading cause of death worldwide by 2020. The disease is chronic and progressive and results in multiple and sometimes protracted interactions with many different healthcare agencies. Throughout the course of the disease, the patient will usually see a primary care physician at the outset, providing the first opportunity for intervention. The new patient-focused UK General Practitioners (GP) General Medical Services contract has encouraged, through direct disease-focused financial incentives (QOF points), a more proactive approach of 'grass roots' COPD disease management, primarily through educating patients at an early stage.

In the UK, the recently published National Strategy for COPD and Asthma will drive, via healthcare commission, improvements in COPD management in primary and secondary care. Primary care providers will be commissioned to screen patients for COPD, perform effective case finding and have quality assured spirometry available to make the correct diagnosis [7].

Can COPD be managed successfully in primary care?

Patients with COPD will spend the vast majority of their time being cared for in the community. The majority of care can be given in this setting; however, there will be times when secondary care facilities and expertise will be required. A small proportion of patients with COPD provide the greatest healthcare burden [8], and it is this group that is often caught up in a 'secondary care carousel', with multiple severe exacerbations and protracted admissions, often complicated by other comorbidities. It is hoped that future therapies will be directed at breaking this inflammatory cycle, ie, those with a 'frequent exacerbator' phenotype. However, the majority of patients can be diagnosed and managed successfully in the community without recourse to hospital-based care. COPD does not often require high-technology, expensive investigations or interventions. The diagnosis is relatively straightforward and drug-based management options are now simple. Preventative therapy (eg, smoking cessation) is usually effective when based in primary care, and with the advent of disease registers, it is feasible to screen asymptomatic smokers who may have preclinical disease. It is also hoped that 'real time' patient-reported outcomes may guide practitioners in identifying disease 'flares', similar to the SMART™ (single maintenance and reliever therapy) approach in asthma.

As the disease progresses, pulmonary rehabilitation programmes can be effectively managed in a community setting; several studies have now shown that acute exacerbations of COPD can be safely and successfully maintained in the patient's own home [9,10]. In addition, general community-based medical practitioners and nurses have the skills to manage COPD and are better placed than secondary care providers to integrate care in a multidisciplinary manner.

A more positive attitude to COPD

Healthcare professionals can sometimes project negative and nihilistic attitudes about COPD. When these feelings are communicated to patients, either consciously or subconsciously, the patients in turn often feel guilty about smoking and that they have caused their own disease. This attitude must be countered and rejected at every opportunity.

Winston Churchill said *"Now this is not the end. It is not even the beginning of the end. But it is, perhaps, the end of the beginning"* [11]. We feel this is an apt quotation to use about the state of knowledge of this terrible disease. Never before has so much attention been focused on this problem, raising the profile of COPD. At every level, from the government to pharmaceutical companies, the degree of interest in COPD has increased, while new drug development is continuing apace. The WHO- and European Union (EU)-backed anti-smoking legislations are getting tighter, sending clear messages to smokers and raising the profile of COPD even further. Levels of research into COPD have never been greater and research output is increasing exponentially. These changes will eventually lead to improvements in care. Moreover, healthcare professionals should be encouraged to review their attitudes and refocus their efforts for each individual patient.

The palliative care approach

At the present time, COPD is not curable. Many patients with COPD, both smokers and nonsmokers, undergo an inexorable decline in health status, ultimately leading to death. Therefore, a major facet of the management of COPD is to acknowledge this fact with patients, help them to understand the disease process and assist them in and dealing with a terminal disease. This can be achieved by adopting a palliative care approach. It is very difficult to identify the terminal phase of COPD for many patients. Indeed, many patients with COPD have poorer QOL scores than those with terminal cancer [12]. Thus, it is even more important to prepare the patients and carers for this time. Treating patients as individuals and helping them to live with COPD until death is not easy. Addressing symptoms can be somewhat easier than dealing with more complicated psychosocial issues. However, all of these concerns must be taken into consideration, and a more holistic approach to care is very much encouraged.

References

1   Hogg JC, Chu F, Utokaparch S, et al. The nature of small-airway obstruction in chronic obstructive pulmonary disease. N Engl J Med 2004; 350:2645–2653.

2   Hogg JC, Macklem PT, Thurlbeck WM. Site and nature of airway obstruction in chronic obstructive lung disease. N Engl J Med 1968; 278:1355–1360.

3   Anthonisen NR, Connett JE, Kiley JP. Effects of smoking intervention and the use of an inhaled anticholinergic bronchodilator on the rate of decline of FEV_1. The Lung Health Study. JAMA 1994; 272:1497–1505.

4   Global Initiative for Chronic Obstructive Lung Disease. Global Strategy for the Diagnosis, Management and Prevention of Chronic Obstructive Pulmonary Disease. December 2011. Available at: www.goldcopd.org/uploads/users/files/GOLD_Report_2011_Feb21.pdf. Last accessed October 2012.

5   US Department of Health and Human Services, Food and Drug Administration. Guidance for Industry. Chronic Obstructive Pulmonary Disease: Developing Drugs for Treatment. November 2007. Available at: www.fda.gov/downloads/Drugs/GuidanceComplianceRegulatoryInformation/Guidances/ucm071575.pdf. Last accessed October 2012.

6   US Department of Health and Human Services, Food and Drug Administration. Guidance for Industry. Acute Exacerbations of Chronic Bronchitis in Patients with Chronic Obstructive Pulmonary Disease: Developing Antimicrobial Drugs for Treatment. September 2012. Available at: www.fda.gov/downloads/Drugs/GuidanceComplianceRegulatoryInformation/Guidances/UCM070935.pdf. Last accessed October 2012.

7   Department of Health. An outcomes strategy for people with chronic obstructive pulmonary disease (COPD) and asthma in England. Available at: www.dh.gov.uk/en/Publicationsandstatistics/Publications/PublicationsPolicyAndGuidance/DH_127974. Last accessed November 2012.

8   Wouters EF. Economic analysis of the confronting PD survey: an overview of results.
    Respir Med 2003; 97(Suppl C):S3–S14.
9   NICE clinical guideline 101. Chronic obstructive pulmonary disease: management of
    chronic obstructive pulmonary disease in adults in primary and secondary care (partial
    update). June 2010. Available at: www.nice.org/uk/nicemedia/live/13029/49397/49397.pdf.
    Last accessed October 2012.
10 Davies L, Wilkinson M, Bonner S, et al. "Hospital at home" versus hospital care in patients
    with exacerbations of chronic obstructive pulmonary disease: prospective randomised
    controlled trial. BMJ 2000; 321:1265–1268.
11 Churchill W. The End of the Beginning. Speech given at the Lord Mayor's Luncheon:
    Mansion House, London; November 10, 1942.
12 Habraken JM, ter Riet G, Gore JM, et al. Health-related quality of life in end-stage COPD and
    lung cancer patients. J Pain Symptom Manage 2009; 37:973-981.

Chapter 2

Epidemiology, risk factors and pathophysiology

Definitions

The term 'Chronic Obstructive Pulmonary Disease (COPD)' is relatively new (see Chapter 1). However, it has now been widely accepted as the worldwide standard term for obstructive airway disease, usually (but not always) caused by tobacco smoke. The Global Initiative for Chronic Obstructive Lung Disease (GOLD) guidelines define COPD as follows [1]:

> *"Chronic Obstructive Pulmonary Disease (COPD), a common preventable and treatable disease, is characterized by persistent airflow limitation that is usually progressive and associated with an enhanced chronic inflammatory response in the airways and the lung to noxious particles or gases. Exacerbations and comorbidities contribute to the overall severity in individual patients."*

This definition provides a better understanding of a complex process by combining the natural history of the condition, the predominant physiological abnormality and the pathological processes involved (Figure 2.1) [2]. COPD is an umbrella term and could be criticised as not being specific enough, as it can apply to other long-term respiratory conditions. It is hoped that, as advances in the understanding of the pathophysiological heterogeneity of COPD (comprising elements of chronic bronchitis, emphysema and small airways disease [3]) are made, we will be able

R. E. K. Russell et al., *Managing COPD*,
DOI: 10.1007/978-1-907673-52-8_2, © Springer Healthcare 2013

to revise the definition of this disease to more accurately reflect the smoking-related condition that practitioners treat.

The major COPD guidelines all have similar definitions of COPD and disease severity classifications (Table 2.1) [1,4,5]. It is worth noting that, although guidelines use lung function as the primary defining parameter in severity classification, only GOLD uses symptoms as well. It is likely that, as we understand more about COPD, new classifications will arise that not only rely on lung function but also take into account symptomatology, possible markers of airway inflammation and systemic features of the disease.

Definition of COPD

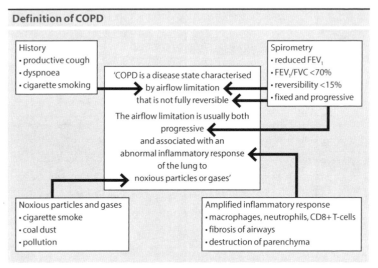

Figure 2.1 Definition of COPD. FEV_1, forced expiratory volume in 1 second; FVC, forced vital capacity. Reproduced with permission from [2]. Copyright © 2004 Taylor & Francis Books UK.

FEV_1 predicted (%)			
Severity	**GOLD**	**ATS/ERS**	**NICE**
I: Mild	≥80	≥80	≥80
II: Moderate	50-80	50-80	50-79
III: Severe	30-50	30-50	30-49
IV: Very severe	<30	<30	<30

Table 2.1 FEV_1 predicted (%). Difference in severity scoring based on lung function. ATS, American Thoracic Society; ERS, European Respiratory Society; FEV_1, forced expiratory volume in 1 second; GOLD, Global Initiative for Chronic Obstructive Lung Disease ; NICE, National Institute for Health and Clinical Excellence. Based on data from [1,4,5].

Epidemiology
The burden of COPD

At present, the global burden of COPD is difficult to determine. Global estimates often rely on data from analyses within limited geographical and socioeconomic areas, predominately from the Western world. Moreover, COPD is still underdiagnosed even within the most efficient healthcare systems, thus underestimating the scale of the problem. The consumption of cigarettes continues unabated [6] and, where this is the case, COPD will inevitably follow. The BOLD (Burden Of Lung Disease) initiative used standardised questionnaires and spirometry to provide global prevalence figures and has found striking differences among countries [7,8].

Mortality

COPD currently ranks as the fifth most common cause of death worldwide [9]. The World Health Organization (WHO) has estimated that by 2020 it will have increased to being the third, making this a global epidemic (Figure 2.2) [2].

COPD is the only common cause of death that has increased in the USA over the past 40 years. At present, COPD accounts for about 30,000 deaths per annum in the UK, which is twice the EU average, and now kills more women in the UK than breast cancer.

Prevalence

The prevalence of COPD is hard to estimate accurately. Approximately 1% of the world's population has COPD. Smokers in the USA have a prevalence of airway obstruction of 14%, which has been corroborated by other studies in the Western world [10], although this value may be higher with more accurate diagnosis using lung function and symptoms [11]. The BOLD study estimated the prevalence of COPD GOLD Stage I or greater to range from 11.4–26.1% [8].

Social costs

Health economic studies of disease and disease interventions collect data on both the healthcare costs of a disease and the indirect costs, such as loss of work and disability. Disability can be measured using disability-adjusted life years (DALYs). This is a measure of time lost from both the disease and any significant disability associated with the disease, and is used to evaluate the effect of various interventions in terms of health-related quality of life (QOL). In 1990, COPD was ranked twelfth of all global disease for DALYs lost, and it has been predicted that by 2020 it will move up to the fifth position (Figure 2.3) [12].

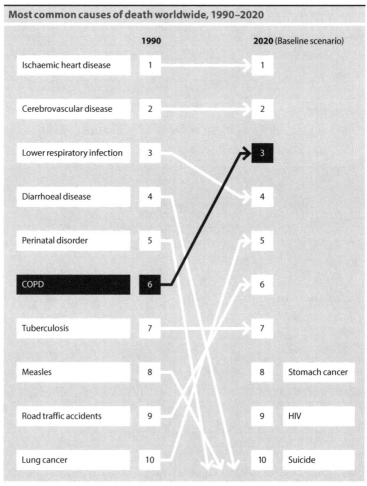

Most common causes of death worldwide, 1990–2020

	1990	2020 (Baseline scenario)	
Ischaemic heart disease	1	1	
Cerebrovascular disease	2	2	
Lower respiratory infection	3	3	
Diarrhoeal disease	4	4	
Perinatal disorder	5	5	
COPD	6	6	
Tuberculosis	7	7	
Measles	8	8	Stomach cancer
Road traffic accidents	9	9	HIV
Lung cancer	10	10	Suicide

Figure 2.2 Most common causes of death worldwide, 1990–2020. HIV, human immunodeficiency virus. Reproduced with permission from [2]. Copyright © 2004 Taylor & Francis Books UK.

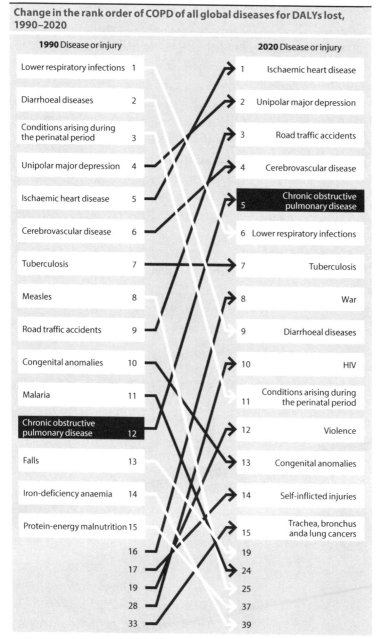

Figure 2.3 Change in the rank order of COPD of all global diseases for DALYs lost, 1990–2020.
Reproduced with permission from [12]. Copyright © 1998 Macmillan Publishers Ltd.

Economic costs

The prevalence of smoking is strongly linked to socioeconomic status [13]. Reducing the overall healthcare burden involves the effective use of both economic and noneconomic measures. Taxation is an obvious choice but could result in the rise of smuggling or black market operations and smokers switching from branded labels to hand-rolled tobacco, potentially leading to increased consumption and risk of unfiltered smoke exposure. Price increases encourage some people to stop smoking and prevent others from resuming the habit or even starting in the first place; adolescents are particularly 'price sensitive' [14]. Noneconomic measures include developing smoking cessation programmes, reducing tar emissions in existing products, countering early nicotine addiction by discouraging young people to smoke, blanket bans on advertising and promotion, and workplace smoking restrictions.

Overall healthcare costs from COPD caused by cigarette smoking can be partially offset by government-raised taxes on tobacco, and in some instances this money can be earmarked for anti-smoking activities [15]. However, by stopping people from smoking, it is possible that healthcare costs may rise, as life expectancy will increase and correspondingly the need for state care.

Many studies have examined the economic burden of COPD. Direct costs (in the years 2000–2004) were found to range from $876 per patient year in the Netherlands all the way to $10,812 per patient year for GOLD Stage III disease in the United States [9].

Risk factors

A variety of risk factors for COPD have been identified (Table 2.2). Clearly, cigarette smoking is the most significant, but others include the effect of diet, early childhood disease and genetic factors.

Smoking

Cigarette smoking is the principal cause of COPD. It is responsible for more than 95% of all cases in the developed world and is increasing in parallel with the increase in COPD in developing countries. A smoking habit can be quantified by calculating the number of pack years a person

Risk factors for COPD
Host factors
Genetic (eg, α_1-antitrypsin deficiency)
Airway hyperresponsiveness: 'Dutch response'
Atopy: mast cell coated with immunoglobulin E and allergen (eg, house dust mite)
Premature baby: small for dates, low birth weight, impaired lung growth
Diet deficient in antioxidant vitamins (A, C and E), fish oil and protein
Gender controversial
Environmental factors
Cigarette, pipe, cigar smoking: tobacco and cannabis
Car exhaust pollution
Industrial pollution: sulphur dioxide particulates <10 mm
Wood fire: biomass fuels
Mining: coal and silica cadmium fumes
Bacterial infection: *Streptococcus* or *Haemophilus*
Influenza virus, adenovirus and HIV

Table 2.2 Risk factors for COPD.

has smoked: 1 pack year = 20 cigarettes daily (1 pack) for 1 year. A significant smoking load is usually around 20 pack years. However, some individuals will be extremely susceptible to the effects of smoking and will rapidly develop progressive disease with minimal tobacco intake. Exposure to passive smoke (environmental tobacco smoke) can be significant in individuals who work in smoky atmospheres (ie, bar workers and entertainers). Ongoing legislation in the Western world to reduce passive smoke exposure will protect these people at work. A 2007 study showed that a no-smoking policy in bars in Dublin significantly improved lung function in bar workers [16].

Cannabis smoking

Smoking cannabis can lead to a COPD-like disease with rapid progression and earlier onset. Often, cannabis is mixed with tobacco. Moreover, the inhalation of marijuana is greater than that of a cigarette, as the smoke remains in the lungs for a longer period of time, leading to increased pulmonary damage. Cannabis has also been shown to cause large apical bullous disease and increased airway inflammation.

Air pollution

Air pollution through the use of biomass fuels leads to bronchitis, and exposure to biomass fuels in poorly ventilated homes is a common cause of COPD amongst women in developing countries [17]. Exposure to sulphur dioxide is also associated with chronic bronchitis.

Genes

In people with the genetic disorder α_1-antitrypsin deficiency, a genetic deficiency of an anti-elastase protein combined with cigarette smoking leads to early and severe COPD. This is a rare cause of COPD (<1%) and no other major genetic factors have been identified. However, it is very likely that multiple genes determine a smoker's susceptibility to developing COPD. Only a minority of smokers who develop COPD fall into this category (~15%), although there is a demonstrable familial tendency of the disease in patients who have early onset disease. Long-term genetic studies involving detailed pedigree data are being conducted. Previous studies suggest a multiple gene effect, with each gene itself playing only a small role. Although there are many reports of genetic association with COPD, few of these findings have been replicated in different populations [18]. Genes implicated include those encoding Serpin E2 [18], tumour necrosis factor-alpha (TNF-α) [19], microsomal epoxide hydrolase [20] and glutathione-S-transferase [21]. Hunninghake et al. [22] have postulated that matrix metalloproteinase (MMP)-12, secreted by macrophages in the air spaces and implicated in the development of emphysema, plays a role in determining lung function and susceptibility to COPD in high-risk groups.

Airway reactivity

The 'Dutch hypothesis' proposes that an allergic mechanism is central to the development of COPD. Orie, in his famous paper of 1961 [23], stated that *"bronchitis and asthma may be found in one patient at the same age but as a rule there is a fluent development from bronchitis in youth to a more asthmatic picture in adults, which in turn develops in bronchitis of elderly patients"*. Of course, we now know that this was, in part, a manifestation of airway remodelling leading to fixed airflow obstruction. Subsequently, this has been supported by the finding of increased levels of airway hyperresponsiveness in some patients with COPD, a risk factor which increases mortality [24] and could be related to increased airway neutrophilia. Could asthma and COPD be part of a spectrum of obstructive airway disease? There is some evidence to support this, although there are many more differences than similarities between the two diseases. However, there are strong arguments against this simple hypothesis, such as the fact that atopy is found in most people with asthma but is not associated with COPD [25].

Diet

Childhood nutrition may play a role in the development of COPD later in life. Babies born with a low birth weight are at increased risk of developing COPD in adulthood. Dietary deficiency of antioxidants has also been proposed to increase the risk of COPD. This hypothesis is attractive for several reasons. There is good evidence that in COPD an oxidant/antioxidant imbalance exists, which may increase tissue inflammation and damage. Antioxidants come (in part) from our diets, so a deficient diet might increase the risk of COPD. Diets rich in fish oil, fresh fruit and vegetables may reduce the risk of developing COPD [26].

Social inequality

COPD is associated with poverty, and there is a much greater prevalence of COPD in lower socioeconomic groups, far more than one would expect even when accounting for smoking prevalence rates. Factors associated with poverty include poor diet, damp housing and more frequent chest infections.

Pathology of COPD

There are characteristic microscopic and macroscopic findings in COPD. When a susceptible individual is exposed consistently to tobacco smoke, changes occur in the airways that are caused by an inflammatory reaction (Figure 2.4) [2]. One could postulate that, given that the first contact cigarette smoke has is with the epithelial lining of the airways and alveoli, this drives a process which ultimately involves a variety of inflammatory cell types, including neutrophils, lymphocytes, macrophages and eosinophils (Figure 2.5) [27]. As a result of aberrant reparative processes

Changes to airways in reponse to exposure to tobacco smoke

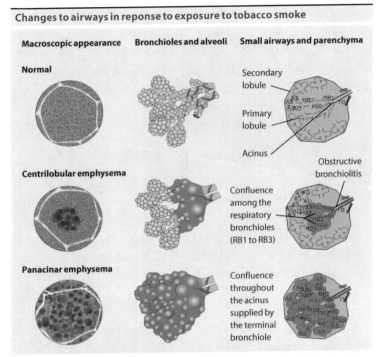

Figure 2.4 Changes to airways in reponse to exposure to tobacco smoke. AD, alveolar duct; AS, alveolar sac; RB, respiratory bronchiole; TB terminal bronchiole. Reproduced with permission from [2]. Copyright © 2004 Taylor & Francis Books UK.

and/or a direct consequence of unchecked oxidative load, lung damage occurs because these cells release proteolytic enzymes that destroy lung connective tissue [28]. This process continues over many years through chronic exposure to cigarette smoke. Damage accrues and becomes irreversible. The microscopic changes lead to larger macroscopic and physiological changes, resulting in disability.

The clinical presentation of COPD manifests itself as a combination of three key pathological processes, all causing different symptoms (Figure 2.6) [2]:

1. Chronic bronchitis, with large airway luminal neutrophilia, increased mucus secretion and reduced clearance secondary to destruction of the mucociliary escalator, together with recurrent viral and bacterial infection and colonisation.

2. Small airways disease, with raised numbers of luminal (CD68+) macrophages and interstitial monocytes/macrophages, and narrowing or stenoses of the bronchioles as a result of fibrosis.
3. Emphysema, with irreversible loss of respiratory units (alveoli) resulting in lack of elastic recoil and reduced surface area for gas exchange.

Although all three processes exist hand in hand, each may have a different pattern of disease with one type of damage being dominant.

Changes also occur to the lung vasculature due to chronic hypoxia, ultimately leading to pulmonary hypertension. This causes ventilation–perfusion inequalities, which exacerbate the breathlessness experienced by patients already breathing at high end-expiratory lung volumes approaching total lung capacity.

COPD also causes systemic effects, and significant changes are seen throughout the body as a whole. These include, weight loss and skeletal muscle weakness, among others. The effects of wasting also increase breathlessness.

Chronic bronchitis

Chronic bronchitis is part of the clinical disease spectrum of COPD; however, many smokers have chronic bronchitis without airflow limitation. It may contribute to the changes in physiology and symptoms seen in patients with COPD (Figure 2.7) [2].

Large airways are lined with pseudo-stratified ciliated columnar epithelia and mucus-producing goblet cells are found throughout these airways. Changes seen in chronic bronchitis include greater amounts of mucus, an increase in the size and number of goblet cells, and larger numbers of macrophages, T-lymphocytes and plasma cells. The submucosal bronchial glands are also enlarged. The mucus hypersecretion that develops may also contribute to airflow obstruction and predispose the patient to lower respiratory tract infections.

Chronic obstructive bronchiolitis

Distal to the bronchi are the bronchioles, which are smaller conducting airways. Inflammation in these smaller airways is sometimes referred

Inflammatory responses to inhaled irritants in COPD airways

Inhaled irritants
(eg, cigarette smoke)

Epithelial cells

Alveolar macrophage

CD8+ lymphocyte

Fibroblast

Neutrophil

IL-8

LTB₄

TNF-α

IL-8

O₂·⁻

O₂·⁻

Connective tissue proliferation and fibrosis

Emphysema

Obstructive bronchiolitis

Proteases

Mucus hypersecretion

LTB₄ inhibitors

Chemokine-, cytokine- and adhesion molecule-directed therapy:
• CXCR2 and CCR2 antagonists
• selectin antagonists
• inhibition of ICAM1, CD11b
• anti-TNF-α
• IL-10

Anti-fibrotic therapy:
• TGF-β1 inhibitors
• FGF inhibitors
• tryptase and PAR2 inhibitors

Alveolar reapir:
• retinoids
• hepatocyte growth factor
• stem cells

Immunosuppressants
CXCR3 antagonists

Antioxidants
iNOS inhibitors

Inhibitors of cell signalling:
• PDE4 inhibitors
• p38 MAPK inhibitors
• NF-κB inhibitors
• PI3K-γ/δ inhibitors
• PPAR-γ agonists

Protease inhibitors:
• NE inhibitors
• cathepsin inhibitors
• MMP inhibitors
• α₁-antitrypsin
• SLPI

Mucoregulators:
• EGF receptor kinase inhibitors
• CACC inhibitors

(See opposite) Figure 2.5 Inflammatory responses to inhaled irritants in COPD airways. Cigarette smoke (and other irritants) activate macrophages in the respiratory tract that release neutrophil chemotactic factors, including interleukin-8 (IL-8) and leukotriene B_4 (LTB$_4$). These cells then release proteases that break down connective tissue in the lung parenchyma, resulting in emphysema, and also stimulate mucus hypersecretion. Cytotoxic T-cells (CD8+) may also be involved in alveolar wall destruction. This inflammatory process may be inhibited at several stages. CACC, calcium-activated chloride channel; CCR, chemokine (C-C motif) receptor; CXCR, chemokine (C-X-C motif) receptor; EGF, epidermal growth factor; FGF, fibroblast growth factor; iNOS, inducible nitric oxide synthase; ICAM, intercellular adhesion molecule; IKK, inhibitors of nuclear factor-kB kinase; IL, interleukin; MAPK, mitogen-activated protein kinase; MMP, matrix metalloproteinase; NE, neutrophil elastase; NF-kB, nuclear factor-kB; PAR, protease-activated receptor; PPAR, peroxisome proliferator-activated receptor; PDE, phosphodiesterase inhibitor; SLPI, secretory leukoprotease inhibitor; TGF, transforming growth factor; TNF, tumour necrosis factor. Adapted from [27].

to as chronic obstructive bronchiolitis and consists of cellular metaplasia and hyperplasia, increased intraluminal mucus, increased wall muscle and fibrosis. These changes ultimately lead to fixed airway narrowing. The presence of increased numbers of pigmented macrophages predates these lesions. Peribronchiolitis is characterised by increased numbers of CD8+ T-lymphocytes. The narrowing of small airways results in airway closure on expiration, resulting in air trapping and hyperinflation.

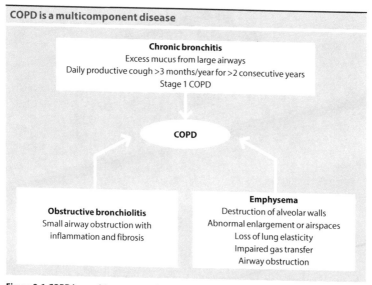

Figure 2.6 COPD is a multicomponent disease. Reproduced with permission from [2]. Copyright © 2004 Taylor & Francis Books UK.

Differences between a normal bronchus and a bronchus in chronic bronchitis

Normal bronchus

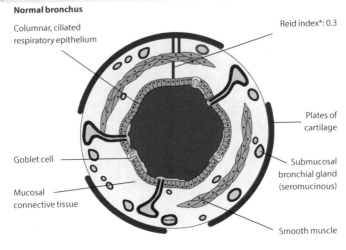

Columnar, ciliated respiratory epithelium

Reid index*: 0.3

Plates of cartilage

Goblet cell

Submucosal bronchial gland (seromucinous)

Mucosal connective tissue

Smooth muscle

Bronchus in bronchitis

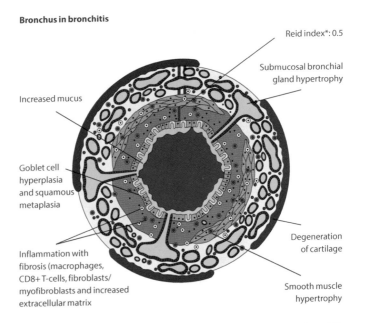

Reid index*: 0.5

Submucosal bronchial gland hypertrophy

Increased mucus

Goblet cell hyperplasia and squamous metaplasia

Degeneration of cartilage

Inflammation with fibrosis (macrophages, CD8+ T-cells, fibroblasts/ myofibroblasts and increased extracellular matrix

Smooth muscle hypertrophy

Figure 2.7 Differences between a normal bronchus and a bronchus in chronic bronchitis.
*Thickness of gland layer to thickness of epithelium and internal cartilage; a normal Reid index is <0.4. Reproduced with permission from [2]. Copyright © 2004 Taylor & Francis Books UK.

Emphysema

It is difficult to appreciate the surface area available for gas exchange in the normal lung using conventional pictures illustrating its gross anatomy. It is not a collection of tubes that slowly get smaller and then end abruptly in an alveolus. In reality, the lung is much more like a very finely pored sponge, containing approximately 300 million alveoli. The area within the lungs that is available for diffusion is 70 m^2, about the same as a tennis court. Each section of lung tissue has a network of pulmonary arteries and veins intimately associated with it — the respiratory bronchiole.

This normal structure is deformed in COPD, and emphysema occurs when the alveoli become enlarged and damaged with loss of elastic recoil. This in turn results in a loss of surface area for gas exchange and ventilatory and perfusion mismatching. It is unclear how this process occurs, although the finding of large numbers of inflammatory cells in emphysematous lungs suggests that the process is an abnormal response to injury. Preservation of the blood supply to terminal lung units is key and occlusion of the terminal bronchioles precedes parenchymal dissolution ('dissolving lung'). Increased stretch forces on existing lung are exacerbated by fracture of the accompanying elastic tissue, a vicious destructive cycle which could explain accelerated lung dissolution seen in some emphysematous patients and backed up by the finding that following lung volume reduction surgery (where stretch forces are increased) lung destruction can actually accelerate. The predominant inflammatory cells are neutrophils, macrophages and T-lymphocytes. The macrophages and neutrophils may be responsible for the release of matrix-destroying enzymes such as neutrophil elastase and MMPs. Experimental animal models have been developed which demonstrate that the instillation and blocking of these enzymes can cause and prevent the production of emphysema, respectively.

At a microscopic level, damage occurs as a consequence of the destruction of boundaries between areas of the lung and the associated breakdown of supportive connective tissue for lung units. This causes airway obstruction and premature airway collapse, which in turn leads to hyperinflation. The loss in respirable area results in diminished gas transfer and breathlessness.

Asthma and COPD

Asthma and COPD are two very different diseases, although severe/chronic asthma has some similarities to COPD. They also may co-exist, leading to a degree of diagnostic uncertainty at initial patient presentation. However, when one considers the definition and pathophysiology of asthma and COPD, the differences become clearer.

Asthma is an airway disease where variable airflow obstruction is a key feature. Asthma often has environmental triggers — the presence of atopy and co-existent allergy is in keeping with a diagnosis of asthma rather than COPD. However, approximately 10% of patients with COPD may have a degree of significant reversibility. Many more demonstrate bronchial hyperesponsiveness, often used as an adjunct to diagnose asthma. Indeed, the severity of bronchial hyperresponsiveness is an independent predictor of improvement in FEV_1 after smoking cessation. The key to differentiating this reversibility is an understanding of the magnitude of change of lung function. Reversibility in asthma may be from a low starting point but should approach normality. In contrast, in COPD there may be reversibility, but it will not approach normality.

At a cellular level, the diseases are also very different. The major cells found in the lungs of patients with asthma are CD4+ T-lymphocytes and eosinophils. The inflammation in asthma can be triggered by allergens, which, through mast cells and dendritic cells in the lung epithelium, leads to the asthmatic inflammatory cascade. In COPD, the trigger is cigarette smoke, which irritates the airway epithelium and airway macrophages, causing a neutrophilic inflammatory response coordinated by macrophages and CD8+ T-lymphocytes with comparatively little mast cell activation.

Asthma may begin early in life and persist or may wax and wane through childhood and adulthood. In contrast, COPD is a disease that has an insidious onset in adult life and is strongly related (at least in the developed world) to cigarette smoke. The breathlessness of asthma is variable and may change with trigger factors and treatment. In COPD, breathlessness is consistent and does not respond to therapy. Sputum production is a common feature of COPD but is uncommon in asthma, whereas the cough in asthma is often nocturnal and dry. Table 2.3 summarises the main clinical differences [29].

Differences between COPD and asthma

	COPD	Asthma
Clinical		
Smoker or ex-smoker	Nearly all	Same as general population
Symptoms under age 45	Uncommon	Usual
Chronic productive cough	Common	Uncommon
Breathlessness	Persistent and progressive	Variable
Inflammatory		
Inflammatory cells	Neutrophils	Eosinophils
	Eosinophils (exacerbations)	Neutrophils (severe asthma)
	CD8+ T-cells +++	Mast cells
	CD4+ cells +	CD4+ T-cells
	Macrophages +++	Macrophages +
Inflammatory mediators	LTB$_4$	LTD$_4$, histamine
	TNF-α	IL-4, IL-5, IL13
	IL-8, GRO-α	Eotaxin
	Oxidative stress +++	Oxidative stress +
Inflammatory effects	Epithelial metaplasia	Epithelial shedding
	Fibrosis ++	Fibrosis +
	Mucus secretion +++	Mucus secretion +
	AHR ±	AHR +++
Location	Peripheral airways predominantly	All airways
	Parenchymal destruction	No parenchymal effects
Response to corticosteroids	±	+++

Table 2.3 Differences between COPD and asthma. AHR, airway hyperresponsiveness; GRO, growth-related oncogene; IL, interleukin; LT, leukotriene; TNF, tumour necrosis factor. Data from [29].

Physiology

As already discussed, COPD is a umbrella term used to describe symptoms produced by several distinct pathologies. The two that contribute most to the physiological abnormality and that are best understood by the general public are chronic bronchitis and emphysema. Indeed, for individuals of a previous generation, the diagnosis of emphysema was thought to be more severe than lung cancer. Perhaps in some ways, they were correct.

Historically, it was fashionable to distinguish between those with bronchitis predominantly and those with emphysema predominantly, known as 'blue bloaters' and 'pink puffers', respectively. The dominant feature of bronchitis tended to be airflow obstruction, whereas patients with emphysema had fewer problems with airflow obstruction and more problems with gas exchange. Of course, for most patients, the reality lies somewhere between the two. Occasionally, however, it is helpful to use these two stereotypes in order to illustrate the physiology of COPD.

Comorbidities

Patients with COPD commonly have other comorbidities which may complicate long-term disease management. Cardiovascular disease is a frequent comorbidity and is the most common cause of death in COPD patients; ischaemic heart disease and heart failure both result from chronic smoking. Diabetes is also prevalent. In addition, there is a four- to five-fold greater risk of lung cancer in patients with COPD compared with smokers with normal lung function. Patients may also suffer from depression (Table 2.4) [30].

Major chronic illnesses present in patients with COPD	
Extrapulmonary disease	**Possible consequences in COPD patients**
Cardiovascular disease	Increased incidence
	Increased dyspnoea (chronic heart failure)
	Reduced physical activity
Cancer (including lung cancer)	Increased mortality
Malnutrition	Increased mortality
	Low fat-free (muscle) mass
	Skeletal muscle weakness
	Increased dyspnoea
	Reduced exercise capacity
Anaemia	Increased dyspnoea
	Possibly increased mortality
Osteoporosis	Fractures
Depression	Increased mortality
Diabetes	Increased respiratory infections
Obstructive sleep apnoea	Sleepiness
	Pulmonary hypertension
	Hypoventilation

Table 2.4 Major chronic illnesses present in patients with COPD. Reproduced with permission from [30].

Assessment
Symptoms

The symptoms of COPD are slowly progressive over many years, in contrast to the episodic and variable symptoms of asthma. Patients have usually lost a considerable amount of their lung volume by the time they present to a doctor, with FEV_1 values often as low as ~50% of predicted. There is usually a history of heavy smoking for many years, often more than 25 pack years.

Progressive shortness of breath on exertion is the predominant symptom, and compensatory behaviour of the patient may delay diagnosis. Dyspnoea results from hyperinflation secondary to small airway narrowing and airway closure as a result of emphysema. This results in a poor QOL, which is further exacerbated by the physical deconditioning resulting from reduced activity (Figure 2.8). Cough and sputum production are common symptoms but are also found in cigarette smokers without airflow limitation (chronic bronchitis). A change in the character of the cough may indicate lung carcinoma. Wheezing may occur during

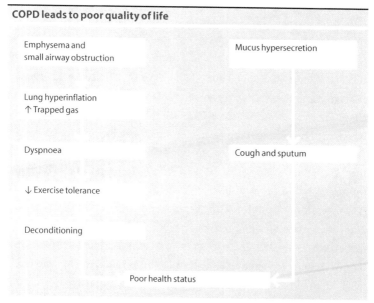

COPD leads to poor quality of life

Emphysema and small airway obstruction

Mucus hypersecretion

Lung hyperinflation
↑ Trapped gas

Dyspnoea

Cough and sputum

↓ Exercise tolerance

Deconditioning

Poor health status

Figure 2.8 COPD leads to poor quality of life.

exacerbations and during periods of breathlessness. Ankle swelling may become noticeable when there is *cor pulmonale* (progressive right-sided heart failure). Weight loss often occurs in advanced disease, but the mechanism is at present uncertain; loss of skeletal muscle bulk may be a response to systemic inflammation.

Signs

When FEV_1 is >50% of predicted, there may be no abnormal signs. The typical patient with more severe COPD shows a large, barrel-shaped chest owing to hyperinflation, diminished breath sounds, distant heart sounds owing to emphysema and prolonged expiration. Patients may also have generalised wheezing on expiration.

Diagnosis

Diagnosis is commonly made from a history of progressive shortness of breath in a chronic smoker and is confirmed by spirometry, which shows an FEV_1/forced vital capacity (FVC) ratio of <70% and FEV_1 <80% of predicted. Staging of severity is made on the basis of FEV_1 (see Table 2.1), but exercise capacity and the presence of systemic features may be more important determinants of overall prognosis. Measurement of lung volume by body plethysmography will show an increase in total lung capacity, residual volume and functional residual capacity, with consequent reductions in inspiratory capacity, representing hyperinflation as a result of small airway closure (Table 2.5) [29]. This results in breathlessness, which may be measured by various dyspnoea scales, and reduced exercise tolerance, which may be measured by a 6-minute or shuttle walking test. Carbon monoxide diffusion is reduced in a proportion of patients, representing loss of respiratory units (emphysema).

A chest X-ray is rarely useful but may show hyperinflation of the lungs and the presence of bullae. High-resolution computerised tomography demonstrates emphysema but is not used as a routine diagnostic test. Blood tests are seldom useful; a normocytic normochromic anaemia is more commonly seen in patients with severe disease than polycythemia owing to chronic hypoxia. Arterial blood gases demonstrate hypoxia and, in some patients with severe disease, hypercapnia.

Lung function test	Result
Forced expiratory volume in 1 second (FEV$_1$; litres)	↓
Forced vital capacity (FVC; litres)	↓
FEV$_1$/FVC (%)	↓
Peak expiratory flow (PEF; litres/min)	↓
Total lung capacity (TLC; litres)	↑
Inspiratory capacity (IC; litres)	↓
Functional residual capacity (FRC; litres)	↑
Residual volume (RV; litres)	↑
Specific airway conductance (sGaw; cmH$_2$O^{-1}.sec^{-1})	↓
Transfer factor for carbon monoxide (T$_{LCO}$; mL/min/mmHg)	↓
Transfer coefficient corrected for alveolar volume (K$_{CO}$ [T$_{LCO}$/V$_A$]; mL/min/mmHg/L)	↓

Table 2.5 Lung function test. Reproduced with permission from [29]. Copyright © 2006 Elsevier.

References

1 Global Initiative for Chronic Obstructive Lung Disease. Global Strategy for the Diagnosis, Management and Prevention of Chronic Obstructive Pulmonary Disease. December 2011. Available at: www.goldcopd.org/uploads/users/files/GOLD_Report_2011_Feb21.pdf. Last accessed October 2012.

2 Hansel TT, Barnes PJ. An Atlas of Chronic Obstructive Pulmonary Disease (Encyclopedia of Visual Medicine Series). London: Parthenon Publishing Group, 2004.

3 Hogg JC. Pathophysiology of airflow limitation in chronic obstructive pulmonary disease. Lancet 2004; 364:709–721.

4 American Thoracic Society and the European Respiratory Society. Standards for the diagnosis and management of patients with COPD. Available at: www.thoracic.org/clinical/copd-guidelines/resources/copddoc.pdf. Last accessed October 2012.

5 NICE clinical guideline 101. Chronic obstructive pulmonary disease: management of chronic obstructive pulmonary disease in adults in primary and secondary care. (partial update). June 2010. Available at: www.nice.org/uk/nicemedia/live/13029/49397/49397.pdf. Last accessed October 2012.

6 Proctor RN. The global smoking epidemic: a history and status report. Clin Lung Cancer 2004; 5:371–376.

7 Buist AS, Vollmer WM, Sullivan SD, et al. The Burden of Obstructive Lung Disease Initiative (BOLD): rationale and design. COPD 2005; 2:277–283.

8 Buist AS, McBurnie MA, Vollmer WM, et al; on behalf of the BOLD Collaborative Research Group. International variation in the presence of COPD (The BOLD Study): a population-based prevalence study. Lancet 2007; 370:741-750.

9 Chapman K, Mannino DM, Soriano DB, et al. Epidemiology and costs of chronic obstructive pulmonary disease. Eur Respir J 2006; 27:188-207.

10 Lindberg A, Jonsson AC, Ronmark E, et al. Prevalence of chronic obstructive pulmonary disease according to BTS, ERS, GOLD and ATS criteria in relation to doctor's diagnosis, symptoms, age, gender, and smoking habits. Respiration 2005; 72:471–479.

11 De Torres JP, Campo A, Casanova C, et al. Gender and chronic obstructive pulmonary disease in high-risk smokers. Respiration 2006; 73:306-310.

12 Lopez AD, Murray C. The global burden of disease 1990–2020. Nat Med 1998; 4:1241–1243.

13 Siahpush M, McNeill A, Hammond D, et al. Socioeconomic and country variations in knowledge of health risks of tobacco smoking and toxic constituents of smoke: results from the 2002 International Tobacco Control (ITC) Four Country Survey. Tob Control 2006; 15(Suppl 3):iii65–iii70.

14 Ding A. Curbing adolescent smoking: a review of the effectiveness of various policies. Yale J Biol Med 2005; 78:37–44.

15 Jha P. Curbing the Epidemic: Governments and the Economics of Tobacco Control. Washington, DC: World Bank, 1999. Available at: www.usaid.gov/policy/ads/200/tobacco.pdf. Last accessed October 2012.

16 Goodman P, Agnew M, McCaffrey M, et al. Effects of the Irish smoking ban on respiratory health of bar workers and air quality in Dublin pubs. Am J Respir Crit Care Med 2007; 175:840–845.

17 Ozbay B, Uzun K, Arslan H, et al. Functional and radiological impairment in women highly exposed to indoor biomass fuels. Respirology 2001; 6:255–258.

18 DeMeo D, Mariani T, Lange C, et al. The SERPINE2 gene is associated with chronic obstructive pulmonary disease. Proc Am Thorac Soc 2006; 3:502.

19 Keatings VM, Cave SJ, Henry MJ, et al. A polymorphism in the tumor necrosis factor-alpha gene promoter region may predispose to a poor prognosis in COPD. Chest 2000; 118:971–975.

20 Sandford AJ, Chagani T, Weir TD, et al. Susceptibility genes for rapid decline of lung function in the lung health study. Am J Respir Crit Care Med 2001; 163:469–473.

21 Cheng SL, Yu CJ, Chen CJ, et al. Genetic polymorphism of epoxide hydrolase and glutathione S-transferase in COPD. Eur Respir J 2004; 23:818–824.

22 Hunninghake GM, Cho MH, Tesfaigzi Y, et al. MMP12, lung function, and COPD in high-risk populations. N Engl J Med 2009; 361:2599–2608.

23 Orie NGM, Sluiter HJ, et al. Bronchitis: an international symposium; April 27–29, 1960. Proceeds published by Royal Van Gorcum, Assen, the Netherlands; 1961.

24 Hospers JJ, Postma DS, Rijcken B, et al. Histamine airway hyper-responsiveness and mortality from chronic obstructive pulmonary disease: a cohort study. Lancet 2000; 356:1313–1317.

25 Barnes PJ. Against the Dutch hypothesis: asthma and chronic obstructive pulmonary disease are distinct diseases. Am J Respir Crit Care Med 2006; 174:240–243.

26 Tabak C, Smit HA, Heederik D, et al. Diet and chronic obstructive pulmonary disease: independent beneficial effects of fruits, whole grains, and alcohol (the MORGEN study). Clin Exp Allergy 2001; 31:747–755.

27 Barnes PJ, Stockley RA. COPD: current therapeutic interventions and future approaches. Eur Respir J 2005; 25:1084–1106.

28 Hogg JC, Chu F, Utokaparch S, et al. The nature of small-airway obstruction in chronic obstructive pulmonary disease. N Engl J Med 2004; 350:2645–2653.

29 Barnes PJ. Chronic obstructive pulmonary disease. In: Laurent G, Shapiro SJ, eds. Encyclopedia of Respiratory Medicine. Boston, MA: Elsevier, 2006; 429–438.

30 Bourdin A, Burgel P-R, Chanez P, et al. Recent advances in COPD: pathophysiology, respiratory physiology and clinical aspects, including comorbidities. Eur Respir Rev 2009; 18:198–212.

Chapter 3

The clinical consultation

Introduction

There are many circumstances where patients may present to a health-care professional in the primary care service (pharmacy, nurse or general practitioner) and be diagnosed with chronic obstructive pulmonary disease (COPD). It might be because of increasing breathlessness or an attack of bronchitis, or the patient might be attending a routine flu vaccination or health screening, or an outpatient (general or specialist) or follow-up clinic after a hospital admission.

Each of these circumstances is a little different and requires a sensitive hand to ask the correct questions and guide the patient through the process of clinical diagnosis, appropriate testing, initiation of treatment and counselling on prognosis. Putting patients on the right clinical track at this stage is important and will be helpful later if and when the disease progresses. Patients are often anxious about seeing a doctor; if the doctor or healthcare practitioner considers this, then it is likely that the consultation will go well and both parties will feel positive about future interactions.

Often patients will have never heard the term COPD before; however, they may suspect they have lung cancer or more commonly emphysema. This is particularly relevant in people over the age of 60 years who have an awareness of air pollution-related deaths and the chronic chest disease health campaigns of the 1950s. On the other hand, they may have been told that they have asthma, which is a familiar disease to many and may be considered by the patient as trivial or less serious. Each patient should have their own individual situation examined and a careful, comprehensive and effective consultation performed.

R. E. K. Russell et al., *Managing COPD*,
DOI: 10.1007/978-1-907673-52-8_3, © Springer Healthcare 2013

The interview

At the outset, it is important to determine why a patient has come and to directly address their concerns. It is vital to establish trust and rapport with these patients, as it is likely that the therapeutic relationship in COPD will be ongoing and may be turbulent.

Symptoms of COPD

Symptoms of COPD that may be evident are presented in Table 3.1. If the patient is seeking help, it is likely that breathlessness will be the predominant symptom. Breathlessness is defined as the abnormal awareness of the act of breathing. In this condition, it is progressive over many years and will occur with less and less activity. The effect of this breathlessness on the patient during certain daily activities, such as the ability to wash, dress and climb stairs, should be recorded. The use of breathlessness scores may be helpful in this regard, eg, the Medical Research Council dyspnoea score [1]. Some patients may not appreciate how disabled they are until questioned. Unfortunately, it is likely that the patient may have lost up to 50% of their

Symptoms of COPD	
Breathlessness	Primary symptom of COPD, often the presenting complaint
	Main source of anxiety and concern of patients
	Often a cause of disability
	Slow onset; is often progressive and may be continuous
	Significantly worse during exacerbations
Breathlessness	Considered normal by many patients as they smoke
	Usually productive; worse in mornings, unusual at night times
Sputum production	Usually white/grey, may be thick and mucoid
	May change colour with attacks of 'bronchitis' (yellow/green)
Past medical history	Wheezing can occur with exertion and as disease progresses
	Chest pain due to an increased effort of breathing
	Chest tightness occurs, especially during exercise
	Weight loss is an important sign both of progressing disease and of other possible problems (eg, lung cancer or tuberculosis)
	Tiredness and lack of energy – may be linked to muscle weakness, depression
	Ankle swelling may indicate progressive right-sided heart failure (cor pulmonale)
	Bloating and early satiety occur with increasing lung hyperinflation

Table 3.1 Symptoms of COPD.

lung function by the time that they present with breathlessness. Thus, there is a great need to consider other, less obvious symptoms.

Coughing with sputum production is often the other predominant symptom. This is often present for many years and is thought of as 'normal' by many smokers. This is not the case, and healthcare professionals should be aware of the need to identify COPD early by addressing these symptoms in particular. Moreover, the occurrence of so-called 'winter bronchitis' in a smoker should raise the suspicion of COPD.

Other symptoms should also be asked about directly. These include chest pain, ankle swelling, weight loss, muscle weakness and wasting. These symptoms are subtle and may not be automatically mentioned by the patient during the consultation. Chest pain can be significant and disabling and it is often caused by the hyperexpansion of the thoracic cavity, causing stretching of the intercostal muscles and ribs. However, in these cases ischaemic heart disease should also be considered. Ankle swelling may be suggestive of *cor pulmonale*. The onset of this has significant implications both for treatment and prognosis. Weight loss is an important prognostic factor in COPD and muscle weakness may occur due to both significant weight loss and the direct effects of the disease on muscles. Finally, do not forget to ask about the patient's mental wellbeing. Depression is a very common finding in COPD and deserves acknowledging and treating [2].

It is possible that the patient may present with other symptoms than those already mentioned. It is important to be aware of the significance of some of these. Cough with haemoptysis, especially in the context of weight loss, is very suspicious of lung cancer. A seasonal variation in symptoms may indicate the presence of asthma. Patients with bronchiectasis produce sputum for most of the year.

Clinical history

An accurate and complete clinical history should be obtained. All of the points mentioned in Table 3.2 should be addressed, not forgetting the importance of taking an occupational history and documenting the patient's current social situation. Attention should be paid to the presence of risk factors. Tobacco smoking is the predominant issue and a smoking history documented using the concept of pack years. Cigars, pipes and cannabis smoking all cause COPD. Occupations that have a great exposure to dust may cause COPD, eg, coal mining. It has more recently been recognised that women are more susceptible to the effects of smoke, both tobacco and from domestic fires (biomass fuel smoke), as causes of COPD [2]. Patients with advancing COPD tend to slip into social isolation, which further exacerbates decline in health and quality-of-life (QOL) status.

It is important to document the exacerbation history of every patient. How many courses of antibiotics and/or steroids have they received in

Complete clinical history	
Patient symptoms	Note down and address them all in order to obtain a complete picture of each individual's pattern of disease
Risk factors	Tobacco smoke, cannabis, other inhaled substances
	Occupation: dusts, chemicals
	Smoke exposure from carbon burning (biomass) fires, domestic and industrial
Smoking history	Age of onset of smoking
	Number of cigarettes a day
	Exposure recorded as pack years
	Previous abstinence, desire to quit
Past medical history	Childhood respiratory disease
	Previous asthma
	Any history of allergic disease (eg, atopy, rhinitis, hay fever)
	Other smoking-related diseases: ischaemic heart disease, peripheral vascular disease, cancer
	Other lung diseases: tuberculosis (active or exposure), pneumonia
Drug history	Current lung treatments
	Pattern of use of antibiotics and/or oral steroids
	Cardiovascular drugs: diuretics, antihypertensives
Social history	Housing
	Occupation
	Family support
	Use of social services
Disease impact	Walking distance (real life outcomes; eg, number of stairs, distance to post box or shops)
	Getting out of house (shopping, day centre, work)
	Need of assistance with normal day-to-day activities
Family history	First-generation relatives might have had COPD or 'chest trouble'
	Other members of family who smoke
	Lung cancer, ischaemic heart disease, peripheral vascular disease, tuberculosis

Table 3.2 Complete clinical history.

the last year? Have they ever been hospitalised with an exacerbation? Have they required any ventilatory support? All of these questions build a fuller picture of the disease impact and the patient's disease phenotype and provide clues to help prognosticate and guide therapy.

Physical examination

A complete examination should be performed. Particular attention should be paid to signs that add prognostic information. These include signs of hypoxia, *cor pulmonale* and cachexia. Table 3.3 lists specific signs to review. However, there may be no abnormal signs in mild COPD and the diagnosis is made on history and lung function testing alone.

Examining the hands may reveal cyanosis and tar-staining of the nails and finger. Clubbing is not found in COPD and may suggest the presence of a lung malignancy or other disease such as bronchiectasis. The hand may flap (tremor), which may mean carbon dioxide retention and could also be associated with a bounding pulse. The pattern of breathing in COPD may be abnormal early on. A prolonged expiratory phase is suggestive of airflow obstruction. The chest wall itself may be hyperexpanded and barrel-shaped. Breathing may require the use of accessory muscles of respiration such as the scalene, trapezius or sternocleidomastoid muscles. The abdominal wall muscles may also be active.

The patient's breathing may be quiet and there may also be crackles present in the lungs. A wheeze is often heard and may lead to diagnostic confusion with asthma. It is essential to remember that many chest diseases can cause an audible wheeze.

Signs of *cor pulmonale* must not be missed and should be specifically sought out. They include a raised jugular venous pulse, an enlarged heart with a loud second heart sound and perhaps even a right heart gallop rhythm. The liver may be enlarged and pulsatile and there may be peripheral oedema present.

Investigations

After taking a clinical history and examining the patient, the diagnosis of COPD will usually be obvious. However, in order to complete the assessment and stage the disease, spirometry is mandatory (can also consider bronchodilator reversibility testing). The differential diagnosis of COPD includes respiratory diseases, which can be difficult to tell apart from COPD on a clinical basis alone (eg, chronic asthma).

Physical examination in COPD	
Breathing	Observe patient breathing at rest for: • comfort; • rate of breathing; • length of expiration; • use of accessory muscles (sternocleidomastoids, trapezius and scalene muscles); • pursed lip breathing; and • abnormal movement of intercostal muscles
Chest shape	Barrel-shaped chest
Hands	Finger cyanosis
	Finger clubbing
	Evidence of smoking (tar staining)
	Increased skin wrinkling
Head and neck	Abnormal venous pulsation (may indicate *cor pulmonale*)
	Central cyanosis
	Hair discoloured by smoking
	Poor dentition
Expansion of chest	Chest hyperexpanded but movement with breathing is reduced
	Movement especially decreased in upper chest
Percussion of chest	May be globally increased
	Loss of cardiac dullness
Breath sounds	Often quiet
	Wheezes may be heard
	Expiratory time is prolonged
Heart sounds	Often quiet and may be inaudible
	Loud second heart sound in pulmonary hypertension
	Tricuspid regurgitation is often heard in *cor pulmonale*
Cachexia	Severe weight loss
	Wasting of muscles: • loss of tibialis anterior (sharp anterior edge to tibia); and • loss of proximal muscle bulk
Other signs	Orthopnoea
	Ankle swelling
	Enlarged liver
	Signs of steroid use – bruising, oral candidiasis, proximal weakness, moon face

Table 3.3 Physical examination in COPD.

Additional tests that should be performed include full blood count, testing for α1-antitrypsin deficiency if age <45 years, serum electrolytes and oxygen saturation if cyanosis is suspected (perhaps followed by formal blood gas analysis). A chest X-ray is essential to both help diagnose COPD and also to pick up other problems, eg, lung cancer. Table 3.4 contains a complete list of tests.

Investigations to consider in COPD	
Spirometry	Mandatory in COPD
	Measures FEV_1 and FVC
	Disease classified by degree of spirometric abnormality
	Consider reversibility testing with bronchodilators if history of asthma, allergy, atopy or significant disease variability
Chest X-ray	Provides a baseline for the future
	Excludes other significant diseases (especially lung cancer)
Full blood count	To look for secondary polycythaemia
	Excludes anaemia as a cause of breathlessness
	Normocytic normochromic anaemia may occur as a systemic feature in severe disease
Electrolytes	Abnormalities can occur in the context of *cor pulmonale*
	Essential before diuretic use
Sputum analysis	Sputum cytology can be helpful if lung cancer is suspected
	Sputum culture helpful during exacerbation
Pulse oximetry	Only provides information on arterial oxygenation
	Affected by changes in peripheral circulation
	Can be used to guide need for full oxygen assessment (arterial blood gas analysis)
Computerised tomography	Increasingly useful in COPD to assess degree of emphysema
	Diagnoses other conditions (bronchiectasis, lung cancer, interstitial lung disease)
	Consider requesting if abnormal or atypical features if chest X-ray abnormal
Electrocardiography	Useful to assess right heart in possible *cor pulmonale*: • prominent p waves; • right axis deviation; and • right bundle branch block
Echocardiography	Useful in assessing degree of pulmonary artery hypertension, tricuspid valve regurgitation and right heart hypertrophy (limited views as emphysematous lung may limit diagnostic views)

Table 3.4 Investigations to consider in COPD. FEV_1, forced expiratory volume in 1 second; FVC, forced vital capacity.

Differential diagnosis

It is important to consider other diagnoses in patients presenting with breathlessness or other symptoms of respiratory disease. Just as it is true to say that 'not all that wheezes is asthma', it is also correct to say that 'not all breathless smokers have COPD'. But of course, many do.

The main differential diagnosis, and the one which causes most confusion, is chronic asthma. The importance of making a clear distinction between COPD and asthma is that asthma therapy can be rather more focused and the practitioner can be more optimistic about prognosis. Other diagnoses to consider include congestive heart failure (CHF), bronchiectasis and even tuberculosis. Table 3.5 clarifies some of the more significant differences in histories and examinations.

Differential diagnosis of COPD

	Age	Symptoms	Sputum	Smoking	Cough	Other	Investigations
COPD	Mid-life	Slowly progressive	++	++	+++	Gradual onset	Irreversible spirometric abnormality
Asthma	Childhood	Variable progressive	–	+/–	++	History of allergy/ atopy, possible family history	Reversible spirometric abnormality
Congestive heart failure	Late life	Persistent	–	+/–	–	Orthopnoea, history of cardiac disease	CXR large heart, increased pulmonary vascular markings
Bronchiectasis	Any	Sub-acute onset	+++	+/–	+++	Recurrent infections, possible childhood disease	CXR or CT scan diagnostic of disease
Tuberculosis	Any		+	+/–	++	Night sweats and weight loss significant	CXR suggestive, sputum analysis diagnostic

Table 3.5 **Differential diagnosis of COPD.** CXR, chest X-ray.

If any symptoms of lung cancer are present, then careful clinical and radiological testing should be conducted.

Ischaemic heart disease and COPD often coexist. A diagnosis can be reached by carefully considering the aetiology of any chest pain and performing an electrocardiography. CHF may present in a similar way to COPD. Knowing the history of longer-term cardiac disease (hypertensive, valvular or ischaemic) can be helpful, as can a chest X-ray. The presence of a raised beta natriuretic peptide can help diagnose cardiac failure and an echocardiogram will document aetiology and degree of cardiac dysfunction.

Many other lung diseases may be confused with COPD. These include primary ciliary dyskinesia, bronchiectasis, obliterative bronchiolitis and even tuberculosis. Each has specific aetiologies and a different balance of symptoms. A careful history of the disease followed by an examination and the right imaging will help to yield a correct diagnosis.

Who should be referred from primary to secondary care?

Referral should occur when a diagnosis is not clear. Where there are symptoms suggestive of lung cancer or tuberculosis urgent referral is mandatory. Where there are symptoms suggestive of lung cancer or tuberculosis, urgent referral is mandatory. Other reasons for referral include early onset of disease (age <45 years), suspected α1-antitrypsin deficiency, suspected *cor pulmonale* and/or the need for oxygen therapy.

Information giving

COPD is a term that is beginning to be understood by the general public. However, individual patients will bring with them their own fears and experiences. They will often feel guilty and have a sense of shame for inflicting the disease on themselves (through smoking). It is helpful to allow them to express these feelings and then draw a metaphorical line through it and put the past firmly in the past.

In order for patients to effectively manage their symptoms, they must have an understanding of the disease process itself. This can often be provided simply by talking through each symptom (eg, cough, sputum production) and explaining the pathological basis for it. For example, explaining hyperinflation to patients and carers is a relatively simple exercise. By asking the patient to take in a deep breath, hold it in, and then take another breath in without exhaling, they can be made to 'feel full of air' (ie, hyperinflated). Breathing tidally following this manoeuvre further adds to this sensation. Many patients feel anxious when this occurs, so simply explaining the phenomena can allay significant fears about their disease. Once patients have some understanding about COPD, they are then in a position to comprehend the treatment options and how they work.

The role of pulmonary rehabilitation can be introduced when discussing what patients can do for themselves. It should be explained clearly that little can be done to improve the lungs themselves; however, it is vital that patients should exercise as much as possible. Preferably, patients should be referred for formal pulmonary rehabilitation.

Prognosis

Patients are coming to practitioners with more knowledge than ever before. In particular, the Internet has enabled patients to access additional resources, making them much more aware about their disease, even though this information can be occasionally misconstrued. The consultation is therefore an ideal opportunity for the practitioner to establish the patient's knowledge base, which is vital when discussing their prognosis. Primary care physicians are greatly skilled in knowing what to say and when, and often have a much better understanding of the background of their patients than secondary care specialists. Patients will want different amounts of information at different times and quite often the information may need to be repeated. Patients have to accept the fact that their lungs cannot be healed.

Exacerbation rates, onset of *cor pulmonale* and the requirement for long-term oxygen therapy are all related to poor prognosis. However, the disease trajectory of COPD is very different to that of cancer, for example, and the slow, gradual decline first shown by the Fletcher and Peto diagram is variable and punctuated by severe and rapid deteriorations, or exacerbations [3]. The latest countrywide data from the UK have demonstrated a 13.9% 90-day mortality rate following admission to hospital with an exacerbation of COPD [4]. Other factors suggestive of a poor prognosis include a low body mass index (<20) and the presence of a low FEV_1 (<30% predicted).

Treatment of COPD exacerbations with noninvasive ventilation may cause difficulties for both patients and practitioners. Patients who have undergone invasive or noninvasive ventilation are often clear about their wishes for the future. Practitioners should not be afraid of asking the question: *'If you required this treatment again would you want it?'*. Very often, patients are candid in their response. Their decision should be documented in such a way so as to be available for admitting teams in the emergency room so that a patient's wishes can be carried out. Living wills and advanced directives are becoming a part of routine clinical practice when dealing with patients with chronic diseases. In order for an advance directive to be valid, it must:

- be made by a person 18 years old or over and has the capacity to make it;
- specify the treatment to be refused (the patient can do this in lay terms);
- specify the circumstances in which this refusal would apply;
- be made by the patient who took the decision under their own volition;
- not have been modified verbally or in writing since it was made;
- be in writing (it can be written by a family member, recorded in the medical notes by a doctor or on an electronic record);
- be signed and witnessed (it can be signed by someone else at the person's direction – the witness is to confirm the signature not the content of the advance directive); and
- include a statement that the decision stands 'even if life is at risk'.

Summary

At the conclusion of a consultation, the patient and practitioner should have discussed:

- symptoms and the effects they have on QOL;
- a history of possible aetiological agents and events; and
- the findings of a physical examination.

A differential diagnosis should be considered and a diagnosis made with suitable tests organised or performed. An assessment and discussion of disease severity and prognosis should be carried out. The patient should leave with as clear a picture as possible about the nature of COPD and have a plan for disease management.

References

1   Bestall J, Paul E, Garrod R, et al. Usefulness of the Medical Research Council (MRC) dyspnoea scale as a measure of disability in patients with chronic obstructive pulmonary disease. Thorax 1999; 54(7):581–586.

2   Han MK, Postma D, Mannino DM, et al. Gender and chronic obstructive pulmonary disease: why it matters. Am J Respir Crit Care Med 2007; 176:1179–1184.

3   Fletcher C, Peto R. The natural history of chronic airflow obstruction. B Med J 1977; 1:1645–1648.

4   Buckingham RJ, Lowe D, Pursey NA, et al. Report of the National Chronic Obstructive Pulmonary Disease Audit 2008: clinical audit of COPD exacerbations admitted to acute NHS units across the UK. Available at: www.rcplondon.ac.uk/sites/default/files/report-of-the-national-copd-audit-2008-clinical-audit-of-copd-exacerbations-admitted-to-acute-nhs-units-across-the-uk.pdf. Last accessed October 2012.

Chapter 4

Management strategies

Guidelines recommend that patients with chronic obstructive pulmonary disease (COPD) should be managed according to the severity of the disease with a stepwise escalation of therapy as the disease progresses (Table 4.1) [1]. It is worth noting, however, that forced expiratory volume in 1 second (FEV_1) is poorly correlated to the level of physical activity, particularly in the early stages of the disease. Breathlessness together with other measures (eg, the BODE index [body-mass index (B), the degree of airflow obstruction (O) and dyspnea (D), and exercise capacity (E)]), may be a better predictor (Figure 4.1) [2].

Anti-smoking measures

Smoking cessation is the only measure shown so far to slow the progression of COPD (Figure 4.2) [3]. However, in advanced disease, stopping smoking has little effect on the underlying chronic inflammation and accelerated decline in lung function. Nicotine replacement therapy (gum, transdermal patch, inhaler) helps individuals to quit smoking, but bupropion, a noradrenergic antidepressant, is somewhat more effective. A novel anti-smoking therapy, varenicline, was approved in the United States and Europe in 2006 [4,5]. It is a partial nicotinic agonist, and in comparative studies, was far more effective than either nicotine replacement therapy or bupropion [4,6]. It is usually given for 12 weeks and may be continued for an additional 12 weeks if necessary. The treatment is well tolerated, and nausea, insomnia, and abnormal dreams are the only significant side effects [4]. Other new anti-smoking therapies,

R. E. K. Russell et al., *Managing COPD*,
DOI: 10.1007/978-1-907673-52-8_4, © Springer Healthcare 2013

GOLD recommendations for therapy at each stage of COPD

Patient category	Nonpharmacologic treatment recommendations	Pharmacologic treatment recommendations
A (low risk, less symptoms)	• Smoking cessation (can include pharmacologic treatment) • Physical activity • Depending on local guidelines: flu and/or pneumococcal vaccinations	• *First choice:* short-acting anticholinergic or short-acting beta2-agonist • *Second choice:* long-acting anticholinergic, LABA, or short-acting anticholinergic + short-acting beta2-agonist
B (low risk, more symptoms)	Same as A, but include pulmonary rehabilitation	• *First choice:* long-acting anticholinergic or LABA • *Second choice:* long-acting anticholinergic + LABA
C (high risk, less symptoms)	Same as A, but include pulmonary rehabilitation	• *First choice:* long-acting anticholinergic or inhaled corticosteroid + LABA • *Second choice:* long-acting anticholinergic + LABA
D (high risk, more symptoms)	Same as A, but include pulmonary rehabilitation	• *First choice:* long-acting anticholinergic or inhaled corticosteroid + LABA • *Second choice:* – Long-acting anticholinergic + LABA, or – Long-acting anticholinergic + phosphodiesterase-4 inhibitor, or – Inhaled corticosteroid + long-acting anticholinergic, or – Inhaled corticosteroid + LABA + long-acting anticholinergic, or – Inhaled corticosteroid + LABA + phosphodiesterase-4 inhibitor

Table 4.1 GOLD recommendations for therapy at each stage of COPD. LABA, long-acting β_2-agonists. Adapted from [1].

such as nicotine vaccines, are in development but have yet to reach the market (see Chapter 6).

Bronchodilators

Bronchodilators are the mainstay of current drug therapy for COPD (Figure 4.3). The bronchodilator response, measured by an increase in FEV_1, is limited in COPD, but bronchodilators may improve symptoms by reducing hyperinflation and therefore dyspnoea. They may also improve exercise tolerance despite the fact that there is little improvement in spirometric measurements. Previously, short-acting bronchodilators,

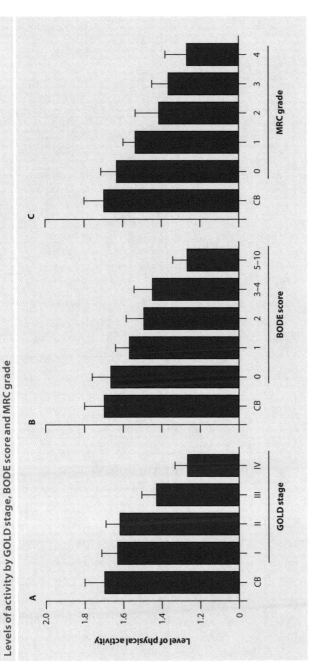

Figure 4.1 Levels of activity by GOLD stage, BODE score and MRC grade. Level of physical activity by Global Initiative for Obstructive Lung Disease (GOLD) stage, BODE (body mass index, FEV₁ for airflow obstruction, dyspnoea, and 6-min walk distance for exercise tolerance) score and Medical Research Council (MRC) dyspnoea grade in 163 patients with chronic obstructive pulmonary disease. Physical activity level ≥1.70: active; 1.40–1.69: predominantly sedentary; <1.40: very inactive. CB, chronic bronchitis. Reproduced with permission from [2].

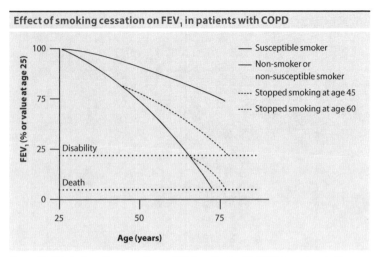

Figure 4.2 Effect of smoking cessation on FEV₁ in patients with COPD. Reproduced with permission from [3].

including β_2-agonists and anticholinergics, were widely used, however, long-acting bronchodilators are now recommended as the preferred therapy. These include the long-acting β_2-agonists (LABAs) salmeterol and formoterol and the once-daily inhaled anticholinergic tiotropium bromide (a long-acting anti-muscarinic antagonist [LAMA]). The new ultra-LABA (uLABA) indacaterol was approved in Europe in 2009 and in the United States in 2011 [7,8]. Indacaterol offers quick onset action and true 24-hour control in both asthma and COPD, with cough being the most frequently reported adverse event. This opens up the way for combination once-daily therapies (LAMAs and uLABAs). As the combination of a LABA and tiotropium also appears to be additive, clinical trials of the combination of these agents are now underway. Although LABAs, LAMAs and inhaled corticosteroids have all been shown to reduce exacerbation rates in patients with COPD by approximately 20%, the cumulative effect of these therapies has not been properly assessed. Two recent 24-week studies evaluated the combination of tiotropium plus inhaled salmeterol and fluticasone versus tiotropium alone (N=743). The combination significantly improved lung function at all timepoints compared with tiotropium monotherapy. However, the mean exacerbation rate was similar between groups [9,10]. Theophylline is also used as an

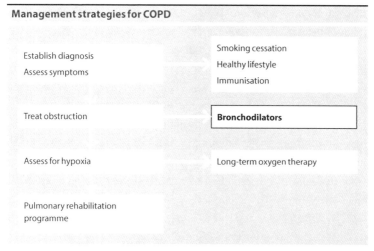

Management strategies for COPD

Establish diagnosis
Assess symptoms

Smoking cessation
Healthy lifestyle
Immunisation

Treat obstruction

Bronchodilators

Assess for hypoxia

Long-term oxygen therapy

Pulmonary rehabilitation
programme

Figure 4.3 Management strategies for COPD.

add-on bronchodilator in patients with very severe disease, but systemic side effects may limit its value. More recently, low-dose theophylline (plasma concentrations of 5–10 mg/L) has been found to reverse steroid insensitivity in COPD and may prove to be a useful addition in the future (see Chapter 6) [11,12].

Exacerbations and the use of antibiotics in COPD

Exacerbations of COPD can be caused by bacteria, viruses or both, with bacteria contributing to 50% of exacerbations [13]. Therefore, antibiotics are often used to treat these exacerbations, but problems surround their use, namely which patients to treat and when, and with what antibiotic.

The National Institute for Clinical Excellence (NICE) COPD guidelines state that antibiotics should be used in patients with COPD with 'a history of more purulent sputum'; those without can be prescribed antibiotics if consolidation (ie, dense areas) is observed on a chest radiograph or there are clinical signs of pneumonia [14]. The use of antibiotics to treat exacerbations in patients with increased cough and sputum purulence and moderate or severe disease is supported by a Cochrane review, which showed that therapy significantly reduced mortality, treatment failure and sputum purulence compared with placebo [15]. There is also evidence to suggest that patients with severe exacerbations are more likely to benefit from antibiotics than those with milder symptoms [16]. Indeed, risk factors for poor outcome identified in various studies include increasing age, severity of underlying airway obstruction, presence of co-morbid illnesses (especially cardiac disease), a history of recurrent exacerbations, use of home oxygen, use of chronic steroids, hypercapnia and acute bronchodilator use. Many of these, of course, reflect increasing disease severity. Furthermore, a study [17] of severe early-onset COPD probands and their relatives found that many of the above predictors were related to the aggregation of exacerbations, suggesting a genetic component to the 'frequent exacerbator' phenotype. Clearly, the 'one size fits all' approach needs to be better quantified when setting goals to avoid treatment failures (Table 4.2) [18].

The NICE COPD guidelines recommend an aminopenicillin, macrolide or a tetracycline as first-line therapy, although input from local microbiologists should be considered [14]. A number of different bacteria have been isolated from the lungs of patients with COPD, including non-typeable *Haemophilus influenzae, Moraxella catarrhalis, Streptococcus pneumoniae*

Goals for treatment of COPD exacerbations	
Goals	**Comments**
Clinical	
Faster resolution of symptoms	Needs validated symptom assessment tools
Clinical resolution to baseline	Needs baseline assessment prior to exacerbation onset for comparison
Prevention of relapse	Relapse within 30 days is quite frequent
Increasing exacerbation-free interval	Needs long-term follow-up after treatment
Preservation of health-related quality of life	Sustained decrements seen after exacerbations
Biological	
Bacterial eradication	Often presumed in usual antibiotic comparison studies
Resolution of airway inflammation	Shown to be incomplete if bacteria persist
Resolution of systemic inflammation	Persistance of systemic inflammation predicts early relapse
Restoration of lung function to baseline	Incomplete recovery is seen in a significant proportion
Preservation of lung function	Needs long-term studies

Table 4.2 Goals for treatment of COPD exacerbations. Reproduced with permission from [18].

and *Pseudomonas aeruginosa* (normally associated with severe airflow obstruction). Attempts have been made to stratify antibiotic use according to the isolated bacteria and host factors, but such approaches have yet to be proven [19]. However, a risk stratification approach is almost certainly advocated using the host factors discussed above.

Vaccination of patients with COPD

The NICE guidelines state that *"pneumococcal vaccination and an annual influenza vaccination should be offered to all patients with COPD as recommended by the Chief Medical Officer"* (Table 4.3) [14,20,21].

Vaccine studies in patients with COPD

Several studies have been performed to investigate the efficacy of *S. pneumoniae* and influenza vaccinations in patients with COPD.

S. pneumoniae

Evidence suggests that pneumococcal vaccination is less effective in patients with COPD than in healthy individuals [22]. Moreover, a Cochrane review concluded that there is no evidence from randomised controlled trials to show that pneumococcal vaccination significantly improves

Vaccination recommendations for patients with COPD
Streptococcus pneumoniae
> 90 serotypes identified
23-valent pneumococcal polysaccharide vaccine (PPV) recommended for defined at-risk groups ≥2 years of age (includes patients with COPD)*
Pneumovax® II is the only licensed PPV in the UK
Vaccine is only effective against serotypes contained in the formulation
Schedule: single dose of 0.5 mL
Influenza virus
Influenza strains included in the vaccine change each year
Annual vaccination is therefore offered between September and early November to those ≥6 months of age in defined risk groups (includes patients with COPD)
Various types of influenza vaccine are licensed in the UK
Schedule (>18 years of age): single 0.1-mL dose

Table 4.3 Vaccination recommendations for patients with COPD. *Serotypes: 1, 2, 3, 4, 5, 6B, 7F, 8, 9N, 9V, 10A, 11A, 12F, 14, 15B, 17F, 18C, 19F, 19A, 20, 22F, 23F, 33F. Data from [20,21].

morbidity or mortality in patients with COPD [23]. However, some studies have shown pneumococcal vaccination to be beneficial. Alfageme et al reported that pneumococcal polysaccharide vaccine was effective at preventing community-acquired pneumonia in patients with COPD who were younger than 65 years of age and in patients with severe airflow obstruction [24]. Additionally, Lee et al demonstrated that the risk of hospitalisation for pneumococcal pneumonia before vaccination was 8.02 compared with controls and 3.87 following vaccination [25].

Influenza

As described in a Cochrane review [26], the number of exacerbations was reduced in patients with COPD who were given the influenza vaccine compared with those who were given a placebo ($P=0.006$). Vaccination caused a significant increase in injection-site reactions, but they were generally mild and transient. Menon et al found that influenza vaccination of patients with COPD is highly effective at preventing acute respiratory illness, particularly in patients with severe disease. It can also significantly reduce the number of outpatient and hospitalisation visits compared with the pre-vaccination period ($P=0.02$) [27].

Oxygen

Home oxygen accounts for a large proportion of healthcare spending on COPD (over 30% in the USA). The use of long-term oxygen therapy (LTOT) is justified by two large trials showing reduced mortality and improved quality of life (QOL) in patients with severe COPD and chronic hypoxaemia (PaO_2 <55 mmHg, 7.3 kPa). These two seminal trials, published within a year of each other, provide the rationale for supplementary O_2 therapy in patients with hypoxaemic COPD [28,29]. More information should be gleaned with respect to oxygen therapy in COPD once the Effectiveness of Long-term Oxygen Therapy in Treating People With Chronic Obstructive Pulmonary Disease (The Long-term Oxygen Treatment Trial [LOTT]) study is complete [30].

The first, larger study [28] was performed in six centres in the USA and Canada and randomised 203 patients with severe COPD (mean FEV_1 30% of predicted) into two groups: one receiving supplementary nocturnal O2 (mean, 12 h/day), the other receiving continuous O2 (mean, 17.7 h/day). Mean follow-up was 19.3 months. Compared with the continuous O2 group, the relative risk (RR) of death in the nocturnal group was 1.94. The subgroups showing a high PaCO2, haematocrit and pulmonary artery pressure or low forced vital capacity (FVC), pH or severe disturbance of mood at entry to the trial appeared to derive the most benefit from continuous O2.

The UK trial [29] recruited 87 patients with severe COPD (FEV$_1$ ~600 mL) and similar profiles to the USA cohort from three centres. In addition, they were all hypercapnic with evidence of congestive cardiac failure (PaCO$_2$ was as high as 8 kPa in one subgroup). The patients were randomised to receive either O$_2$ for 15 h/day or no O$_2$ and were followed for 5 years. The RR was lower than the American trial at 1.49 in favour of supplementary O$_2$ largely because, in the 66 male patients, the survival curves did not start to separate until the 500th day. In the small group of women (n=21; 12 receiving no O$_2$, 9 supplemented with O$_2$), the RR at 3 years was a very high 6.1 in favour of supplementary O$_2$, with the effects becoming immediately apparent. It is unfortunate that this observation was never followed up, although the magnitude of the effect may have been grossly exaggerated by the small sample size. As in the American study, it was speculated that rising PaCO$_2$ and red cell mass levels could predict mortality.

It is clear that supplementary O$_2$ improves survival in hypoxaemic patients (PaO$_2$ ~6.8 kPa) with COPD and evidence of right heart failure. However, the role of pulmonary hypertension in COPD is an emerging field. Recently, it has become clear that fibrosis with emphysema often results in early and severe pulmonary hypertension. It is unclear whether this is a separate disease entity, an isolated feature of idiopathic pulmonary fibrosis or a combination of both processes.

More recent studies have demonstrated that patients with less severe hypoxaemia do not appear to benefit from O$_2$ supplementation. Therefore, the selection of patients is important when prescribing this expensive therapy. Similarly, treatment of nocturnal hypoxaemia does not appear to be beneficial in terms of survival or delaying the use of LTOT in patients with COPD.

Corticosteroids

Inhaled corticosteroids are now the mainstay of chronic asthma therapy, and the recognition that chronic inflammation is also present in COPD provided a rationale for their use in COPD. Indeed, inhaled corticosteroids are now prescribed widely in the treatment of COPD, even though they are only approved for patients with an FEV_1 <50% of predicted (60% for seretide) with two or more exacerbations per year. There is no effect of inhaled corticosteroids on all-cause mortality in COPD. The inflammation in COPD shows little or no suppression even with the use of high doses of inhaled or oral corticosteroids. This may reflect the fact that neutrophilic inflammation is not suppressible by corticosteroids. Indeed, neutrophil survival is prolonged by steroids. There is also evidence for an active cellular resistance to corticosteroids, with no evidence that even high doses suppress the synthesis of inflammatory mediators or enzymes. This is related to decreased activity and expression of histone deacetylase-2 (HDAC2), which is required for corticosteroids to switch off activated inflammatory genes, such as those encoding tumour necrosis factor (TNF)-α, interleukin (IL)-8 and matrix metalloproteinase (MMP)-9.

Approximately 10% of patients with stable COPD show some symptomatic and objective improvement with oral corticosteroids. These patients may have concomitant asthma, as both diseases are very common. Furthermore, they have elevated sputum eosinophils (>3%) and exhaled nitric oxide, which are features of asthmatic inflammation. Long-term treatment with high doses of inhaled corticosteroids fails to reduce disease progression, even at the early stages of the disease. However, there is a small protective effect against acute exacerbations in patients with severe disease (~20% reduction). There is also a small beneficial effect of systemic corticosteroids in treating acute exacerbations of COPD, with a reduction in the risk of treatment failure (NNT 10) and rate of relapse within a month of treatment with corticosteroid treatment, as well as a reduced length of hospital admission (mean reduction 1.22 days) [31]. The reasons for this discrepancy between steroid responses in acute versus chronic COPD may relate to differences in the inflammatory response (increased eosinophils) or airway oedema in exacerbations.

Combination inhalers

Inhalers that combine a LABA and a corticosteroid, such as formoterol/ budesonide and salmeterol/fluticasone, may be more effective than either component alone and are now commonly used in patients with COPD. It is common to start patients off on tiotropium once daily and then to add a combination inhaler for patients with more severe disease who have frequent exacerbations, rather than using an inhaled corticosteroid alone.

Other drug therapies

Systematic reviews show that mucolytic therapies reduce exacerbations, yet most of the benefit (nearly a 30% reduction) appears to come from data involving N-acetylcysteine (NAC), a thiol that is also an antioxidant. The standard dose of 600 mg once daily is probably not high enough given its low bioavailability and short half-life (6 hours), and perhaps doses of 1200-1600 mg are needed. An alternative to NAC is its lysine salt nacystelyn (NAL), which is a more potent antioxidant and has a neutral pH in solution, thereby making it more amenable to the patient via the inhaled route. A related thiol and mucolytic, erdosteine, is now licensed in the UK for the treatment of COPD, and may improve QOL in addition to reducing exacerbations [32]. It is worth noting that when selecting patients with COPD for trials involving mucolytics, any concomitant use of inhaled steroids may reduce the overall positive effects.

Interest in statins as an adjunct for the treatment of COPD has gathered pace. Given their pleiotropic effects on matrix remodelling, oxidant load and inflammation within the lung, statins may be useful therapies. However, more specific patient outcome trials need to be conducted. Interestingly, a 2008 trial in 125 patients with stable COPD showed a significant improvement in exercise time with pravastatin compared with placebo [33].

There is no concrete evidence that cysteinyl leukotriene antagonists, such as montelukast, are beneficial in COPD, although they are sometimes used in combination with other treatments (eg, bronchodilators) if it is felt that there is an asthmatic component to a patient's airway disease. Opiates, such as codeine, may reduce dyspnoea in patients with COPD and help suppress cough if used short-term, but this minimal benefit is outweighed by their side effects, such as constipation and psychological dependence. Low-dose morphine sulphate may be particularly beneficial against extreme dyspnoea in patients with end-stage disease. Additional palliative therapies will be discussed in Chapter 5.

Noninvasive ventilation

Noninvasive positive pressure ventilation (NIPPV) uses a simple nasal mask and thus avoids the need for endotracheal intubation. It reduces the need for mechanical ventilation in acute exacerbations of COPD in hospital by correcting acidosis at an early stage. Domiciliary NIPPV may improve oxygenation and reduce hospital admissions in patients with severe COPD and hypercapnia. In a 2-year trial in 66 patients with COPD, treatment with NIPPV plus rehabilitation led to greater improvements in pulmonary function, gas exchange, exercise tolerance, and QOL over the long term than rehabilitation alone [34].

Pulmonary rehabilitation

Pulmonary rehabilitation consists of a structured programme of education, exercise and physiotherapy and has been shown in controlled trials to improve the exercise capacity and QOL of patients with severe COPD, with a reduction in health-care utilisation and hospitalisation. Pulmonary rehabilitation is now an important part of the management plan in patients with severe COPD.

Nurse-led strategies

Reducing the number of inpatient bed days is vitally important for patients with COPD. This is best achieved using a multidisciplinary approach via a nurse-led COPD outreach service and outpatient follow-up service. Regular team meetings provide the opportunity to close the care loop and give support to team members.

Lung volume reduction

Surgical removal of emphysematous lung improves ventilatory function in carefully selected patients. The reduction in hyperinflation improves the mechanical efficiency of the inspiratory muscles. Careful patient selection after a period of pulmonary rehabilitation is essential. Patients with localised upper lobe emphysema with poor exercise capacity do best, but there is a relatively high operative mortality, particularly for patients who have a low diffusing capacity. Significant functional improvements include:

- increased FEV_1;
- reduced total lung capacity and functional residual capacity;
- improved function of respiratory muscles;
- improved exercise capacity; and
- improved QOL.

Benefits persist for at least a year in most patients, but careful long-term follow-up is needed in order to evaluate the long-term benefits of this therapy.

Nonsurgical bronchoscopic lung volume reduction has been achieved by insertion of one-way valves using fibre optic bronchoscopy. This gives significant improvement in some patients and appears to be safe, but collateral ventilation reduces the efficacy of this treatment so that significant deflation of the affected lung may not be achieved. A number of other bronchoscopic treatments for emphysema are under development, including airway bypass techniques, bronchial, spigots, and lung volume reduction coils [35,36].

Lung transplantation

Long-term results of lung transplantation are limited by significant complications that impair survival. Survival rates of approximately 80% at 1 year, 50% at 5 years and 35% at 10 years have been reported. Bronchiolitis obliterans is the most important long-term complication of lung transplantation, resulting in decreased pulmonary function. In general, a patient with COPD can be considered an appropriate candidate for transplantation when the FEV_1 is below 25% of predicted and/or the $PaCO_2$ is >55 mmHg. Bilateral lung transplantation is preferable in patients with COPD who have chances of better long-term survival. Single lung transplantation is better suited to pulmonary fibrosis, although the availability of donor organs is variable.

References

1 Global Initiative for Chronic Obstructive Lung Disease. Global Strategy for the Diagnosis, Management and Prevention of Chronic Obstructive Pulmonary Disease. December 2008. December 2011. Available at: www.goldcopd.org/uploads/users/files/GOLD_Report_2011_Feb21.pdf. Last accessed October 2012.

2 Bourdin A, Burgel P-R, Chanez P, et al. Recent advances in COPD: pathophysiology, respiratory physiology and clinical aspects, including comorbidities. Eur Respir Rev 2009; 18:198-212.

3 Fletcher C, Peto R. The natural history of chronic airflow obstruction. Br Med J 1977; 1:1645–1648.

4 Chantix [package insert]. New York, NY: Pfizer Inc; 2011.

5 European Medicines Agency. Summary of product characteristics for CHAMPIX. Available at: www.ema.europa.eu/docs/en_GB/document_library/EPAR_-_Product_Information/human/000699/WC500025251.pdf. Last accessed October 2012.

6 Aubin HJ, Bobak A, Britton JR, et al. Varenicline versus transdermal nicotine patch for smoking cessation: results from a randomised open-label trial. Thorax 2008; 63:717-724.

7 European Medicines Agency. Summary of product characteristics for Onbrez Breezhaler. Available at: www.ema.europa.eu/docs/en_GB/document_library/EPAR_-_Product_Information/human/001114/WC500053732.pdf. Last accessed October 2012.

8 Arcapta Neohaler [package insert]. East Hanover, NJ: Novartis Pharmaceuticals Corporation; 2011.

9 Park KS, Park HY, Park SY, et al. Comparison of tiotropium plus fluticasone propionate/salmeterol with tiotropium in COPD: a randomized controlled study. Respir Med 2012; 106:382-389.

10 Hanania NA, Crater GD, Morris AN, et al. Benefits of adding fluticasone propionate/salmeterol to tiotropium in moderate to severe COPD. Respir Med 2012; 106:91-101.

11 Cosio BG, Iglesias A, Rios A, et al. Low-dose theophylline enhances the anti-inflammatory effects of steroids during exacerbations of COPD. Thorax 2009; 64:424-429.

12 Ford PA, Durham AL, Russell REK, et al. Treatment effects of low-dose theophylline combined with an inhaled corticosteroid in COPD. Chest 2010; 137:1338-1344.

13 Sethi S. The problems of meta-analysis for antibiotic treatment of chronic obstructive pulmonary disease, a heterogeneous disease: a commentary on Puhan et al. BMC Med 2008; 6:29.

14 NICE clinical guideline 101. Chronic obstructive pulmonary disease: management of chronic obstructive pulmonary disease in adults in primary and secondary care. (partial update). June 2010. Available at: www.nice.org/uk/nicemedia/live/13029/49397/49397.pdf. Last accessed October 2012.

15 Ram FS, Rodriguez-Roisin R, Granados-Navarrete A, et al. Antibiotics for exacerbations of chronic obstructive pulmonary disease. Cochrane Database Syst Rev 2006; 2:CD004403.

16 Soto FJ, Varkey B. Evidence-based approach to acute exacerbations of COPD. Curr Opin Pulm Med 2003; 90:117–124.

17 Foreman MG, DeMeo DL, Hersh CP, et al. Clinical determinants of exacerbations in severe, early-onset COPD. Eur Respir J 2007; 30:1124-1130.

18 Barnes PJ, Drazen JM, Rennard SI, et al, eds. Asthma and COPD. Basic Mechanisms and Clinical Management. London, UK: Elsevier, 2009.

19 Anzueto A, Sethi S, Martinez FJ. Exacerbations of chronic obstructive pulmonary disease. Proc Am Thorac Soc 2007; 4:554–564.

20 Salisbury D, Ramsay M, Noakes K (eds). Pneumococcal. In: Immunisation against infectious disease. London, UK: Department of Health and The Stationery Office, 2012;295-313.

21 Salisbury D, Ramsay M, Noakes K (eds). Influenza. In: Immunisation against infectious disease. London, UK: Department of Health and The Stationery Office, 2012;185-216.

22 Schenkein JG, Nahm MH, Dransfield MT. Pneumococcal vaccination for patients with COPD: current practice and future directions. Chest 2008; 133:767–774.

23 Granger R, Walters J, Poole PJ, et al. Injectable vaccines for preventing pneumococcal infection in patients with chronic obstructive pulmonary disease. Cochrane Database Syst Rev 2006; 4:CD001390.

24 Alfageme I, Vazquez R, Reyes N, et al. Clinical efficacy of anti-pneumococcal vaccination in patients with COPD. Thorax 2006; 61:189–195.

25 Lee TA, Weaver FM, Weiss KB. Impact of pneumococcal vaccination on pneumonia rates in patients with COPD and asthma. J Gen Intern Med 2007; 22:62–67.

26 Poole PJ, Chacko E, Wood-Baker RW, et al. Influenza vaccine for patients with chronic obstructive pulmonary disease. Cochrane Database Syst Rev 2006; 1:CD002733.

27 Menon B, Gurnani M, Aggarwal B. Comparison of outpatient visits and hospitalisations, in patients with chronic obstructive pulmonary disease, before and after influenza vaccination. Int J Clin Pract 2008; 62:593–598.

28 Nocturnal Oxygen Therapy Trial Group. Continuous or nocturnal oxygen therapy in hypoxemic chronic obstructive lung disease: a clinical trial. Ann Intern Med 1980; 93:391-398.

29 Report of the Medical Research Council Working Party. Long term domiciliary oxygen therapy in chronic hypoxic cor pulmonale complicating chronic bronchitis and emphysema. Lancet 1981; 317:681-686.

30 Effectiveness of Long-term Oxygen Therapy in Treating People With Chronic Obstructive Pulmonary Disease (The Long-term Oxygen Treatment Trial [LOTT]). www.clinicaltrials.gov/ct2/show/NCT00692198. ClinicalTrails.gov, A service of the U .S. National Institutes of Health. Updated April 23, 2012. Accessed November 2012.

31 Walters JAE, Gibson PG, Wood-Baker R, et al. Systemic corticosteroids for acute exacerbations of chronic obstructive pulmonary disease. Cochrane Database Syst Rev 2009; 1:CD001288.

32 Moretti M, Bottrighi P, Dallari R, et al; EQUALIFE Study Group. The effect of long-term treatment with erdosteine on chronic obstructive pulmonary disease: the EQUALIFE Study. Drugs Exp Clin Res 2004; 30:143-152.

33 Lee TM, Lin MS, Chang NC. Usefulness of C-reactive protein and interleukin-6 as predictors of outcomes in patients with chronic obstructive pulmonary disease receiving pravastatin. Am J Cardiol 2008; 101:530-535.

34 Duiverman ML, Wempe JB, Bladder G, et al. Two-year home-based nocturnal noninvasive ventilation added to rehabilitation in chronic obstructive pulmonary disease patients: a randomized controlled trial. Respir Res 2011; 12:112.

35 Gasparini S, Zuccatosta L, Bonifazi M, et al. Bronchoscopic treatment for emphysema: state of the art. Respiration 2012; 84:250-263.

36 Slebos D-J, Klooster K, Ernst A, et al. Bronchoscopic lung volume reduction coil treatment of patients with severe heterogeneous emphysema. Chest 2012; 142:574-582.

Chapter 5

Palliative care in COPD

The annual death rate in the UK from chronic obstructive pulmonary disease (COPD) approaches that of lung cancer [1]. Palliative care in this group of patients is challenging in terms of the assessment and provision of their emotional, physical, psychological, spiritual and social needs and cares. Palliative care is the active holistic care of patients with advanced progressive illness. It includes management of pain and other symptoms and provision of psychological, social and spiritual support. The goal is the achievement of the best possible quality of life for patients and their families. Many aspects are applicable earlier in the course of the illness in conjunction with other treatments [2]. COPD brings with it a multitude of physical, emotional, social and psychological symptoms and the consequent end-of-life symptom management, prognostication, communication, service planning and delivery aspects. Patients with COPD have significant end-of-life needs, but are much less likely than patients with cancer to access or receive appropriate palliative care [3]. Predicting prognosis in COPD is difficult due to the variable illness trajectory [1], with the gradual decline over a number of years with acute exacerbations which may or may not be fatal. In a subgroup of patients, COPD can be a relentlessly progressive disease even when they have stopped smoking. Patients invariably reach a point at which they will require palliative interventions. Dyspnoea is the most distressing symptom experienced by these patients, which in the later stages of the disease becomes 'refractory' or not responsive to traditional dyspnoea management. The focus of care then shifts to relieving symptoms. Many pharmacological and nonpharmacological interventions can help with this, including oxygen, opioids, psychotropic drugs, inhaled furosemide, heliox, rehabilitation,

R. E. K. Russell et al., *Managing COPD*,
DOI: 10.1007/978-1-907673-52-8_5, © Springer Healthcare 2013

nutrition, psychosocial support, breathing techniques and breathlessness clinics (Table 5.1).

The 'End of Life Care Strategy' in the UK [4] advocates the use of end of life tools such as the Gold Standards Framework, Liverpool Care Pathway, Preferred Priorities for Care and the process of Advance Care Planning (ACP) across all disease groups. The focus away from just cancer palliative care is welcome but still brings its own challenges for palliative care for patients with COPD.

Symptom burden

Skilbeck et al [5] looked at 63 patients with COPD over the age of 55 years who had been admitted to hospital with an exacerbation in the preceding 6 months. Breathlessness was the most significant debilitating symptom, reported in 95% of patients, with 60% reporting severe symptoms. Other common symptoms included pain, fatigue, difficulty sleeping and thirst as well as decreased physical, social and emotional functioning. Other studies have compared the care of patients with end-stage COPD with that of patients with lung cancer. Gore et al [6] compared 50 patients with severe COPD with 50 patients with inoperable non-small cell lung cancer. The study assessed quality of life (QOL) as well as the quantity and quality of medical and social care received. The results showed that patients with COPD had worse QOL

Palliative interventions for refractory dyspnoea		
Oxygen	**Pharmacological**	**Nonpharmacological**
Hypoxaemic*	Opioids	Rehabilitation*
Nonhypoxaemic†	• oral*	Nutrition‡
	• parenteral*	Psychosocial support‡
	• inhaled†	Breathing techniques*
	Psychotropic drugs	• positioning
	• anxiolytics‡	• pursed lip breathing
	• phenothiazines†	Breathlessness clinics‡
	• selective serotonin reuptake inhibitors‡	
	Inhaled furosemide‡	
	Heliox‡	

Table 5.1 Palliative interventions for refractory dyspnoea. *Evidence generally supports use of intervention for the management of refractory dyspnoea in COPD. †Current available evidence does not support use of this intervention. ‡Further investigation required.

scores than those in the lung cancer group. They also demonstrated an increase in depressive symptoms over that of the lung cancer group, using the depression subscales of the Hospital Anxiety and Depression Scale (HADS). Activity levels in the COPD group were also lower; 82% were housebound, compared with 36% of patients in the lung cancer group. None of the patients with COPD were offered palliative care. In general, the patients with COPD felt worse than the patients with lung cancer, because even though the two groups have similar symptoms, they did not have access to comparable healthcare input. This could lead to feelings of hopelessness and guilt.

Lokke et al [7] showed that many smokers develop airway obstruction if they live long enough and continue to smoke, and that the number who do so increases because of a decline in competing mortality. Of the continuous smokers studied, at least 25% had COPD, more than the previous estimates of about 15%.

As we have already described, the GOLD guidelines recommend a stepwise approach to care as lung function declines and patients become more symptomatic, involving many different therapies including bronchodilators, pulmonary rehabilitation, inhaled glucocorticoids and oxygen.

Advance Care Planning for patients with COPD in the UK

"Advance care planning is a voluntary process of discussion and review to help an individual who has capacity to anticipate how their condition may affect them in the future and, if they wish, set on record: choices about their care and treatment and/or an advance decision to refuse a treatment in specific circumstances, so that these can be referred to by those responsible for their care or treatment (whether professional staff or family carers) in the event that they lose capacity to decide once their illness progresses" [8].

The UK Department of Health End of Life Strategy [4] advocates that all patients with an advanced life-limiting illness will be able to participate in Advance Care Planning (ACP). In the UK, this takes place in the anticipation of deterioration in the future and attendant loss of capacity to make decisions or communicate. ACP may include a Statement of Preferences and Wishes (eg, Preferred Priorities for Care) and/or an Advance Decision to Refuse Treatment (ADRT). Consideration may also need to be given to Lasting Power of Attorney (Personal Welfare) and the Best Interests principles.

A review of the ACP literature by the Royal College of Physicians [9] identified that 60–90% of the general public was broadly supportive of ACP. The majority of individuals were happy to discuss ACP when their condition was stable and discussions with patients with long-term conditions or as part of an end-of-life management plan increased patient satisfaction. However, ACP may be a series of conversations rather than just one. Information and planning needs/perceptions of patients may change during the course of their illness. Cultural issues may also influence the desire to take part in ACP conversations [10].

A review of barriers to ACP by Gott et al reported that such discussions are rarely initiated. There is inadequate information provision about the course of COPD at diagnosis, a lack of consensus about who should initiate discussions and in what setting they should take place, and a lack of understanding or definition of what 'end of life' means in COPD [11]. Caution should be taken with using a 'one-size-fits-all' approach in COPD. A study by Jones et al [12] of the needs of patients dying from COPD indicated that patients desired better education and information about their condition, but information needs were variable and patients were sometimes unwilling to contemplate the future. Similarly Schwartz discusses the phenomenon of 'response shift', the process whereby in the face of severe disease or impending death, individuals abandon their usual 'roadmap' of values and adapt new perspectives [13]. These shifts can make the application of 'black-and-white' advance planning processes inappropriate, as patient's preferences and wishes may change.

There is also consensus that one form of documentation may not suit all patients [9]. It is important for health and social care staff to be confident and competent in the ACP to facilitate and enable the process, create the documentation and liaise with other health and social care professionals in order to implement patients' preferences and wishes. Couceiro and Pandiellla report that ACP increases the quality of decisions at the end of life of the patients with COPD [14].

Good communication is a key part of the patient, family and healthcare professional interaction [10]. There should be information available about treatments, medications and rehabilitation strategies, as well as making and supporting the consequences of difficult conversations during and at the end of life. The seminal work by Glaser and Strauss [15] highlighted the importance of communication in serious illness or terminal care. We know from work done in communication with patients with cancer that effective communication skills positively influence the rate of patient recovery, effective pain control, adherence to treatment regimens and psychological functioning. Ineffective skills lead to reluctance to disclose important issues or feelings, poor patient compliance with treatment regimens, increased healthcare professional stress, lack of job satisfaction and emotional burnout.

The challenge and uncertainty of prognostication and identifying the final days or weeks of a patient's life is widely reported and has been said to lead to *"prognostic paralysis has been described, whereby clinicians of patients with uncertain illness trajectories prevaricate when considering end-of-life issues"* [16]. Specific barriers to communicating with patients with COPD include difficulty in prognostication, disease trajectory and willingness to discuss [17]. Specific patient barriers also exist, such as the housebound nature of patients with COPD who are oxygen-dependent, uncertain of continuity of care and who would look after them at the time of death. Other symptoms, such as increased depression, could lead to patients viewing communication interactions poorly and may influence their end-of-life treatment choices and preferences, such as noninvasive ventilation or resuscitation. A review of recent research activity in palliative care and COPD reports the importance of ACP and improving communication as an important opportunity to improve the quality of end-of-life care in patients with COPD [18]. Increasingly, studies looking at the communication needs of patients with COPD have found the value and importance of good communication.

Discussing Advance Care Planning

Bevan et al report the general points to consider when discussing ACP [10]. Practitioners may have an understanding of the typical physical course of COPD, but a patient's perspective or experience may be different and as such they may or may not be ready to discuss in detail physical deterioration or preferences and wishes for care. The content of the conversations may vary and range from considerations of preferences and wishes to more formal decisions such as an Advance Decision to Refuse Treatment. The context of the conversation may influence the content, eg, admission or discharge from hospital, transfer to a nursing home or the withdrawal of longstanding management. Some conversations may consider future events (such as readmission to hospital or not), while others may be crisis conversations with little time to build rapport and trust. The confidence and competence of the healthcare professional facilitating the conversation may also influence its content and the decision making. A list of resources on the subject of ACP are listed in Table 5.2.

Advance care planning resources in the United Kingdon
Patient resources
Planning For Your Future Care: A Guide   www.endoflifecareforadults.nhs.uk/publications/planningforyourfuturecare   Guide educating patients about advance care planning (ACP)
Advance Decision to Refuse Treatment (ADRT) proforma   www.endoflifecareforadults.nhs.uk/publications/adrtform   Patient template for writing an ADRT
Dying Matters Resources   www.dyingmatters.org/page/dying-matters-leaflets   Leaflet 1: 'Five Things to do before I die'   Leaflet 2: 'One last thing...'   Leaflet 3: 'I could do with a chat'   Leaflet 4: 'Someone you know is bereaved'   Leaflet 5: 'To do list'   Leaflet 6: 'Remember when we...'   Leaflet 7: 'Thinking of you...'   Leaflet 8: 'Talking to children about dying'   Leaflet 9: 'Putting your house in order'   Leaflet 10: 'Myth busting'   Leaflet 11: 'Time to talk?'   Website aimed at the general public and professionals increasing awareness of dying
Preferred Priorities for Care   www.endoflifecareforadults.nhs.uk/tools/core-tools/preferredprioritiesforcare   Example of a statement of preferences and wishes
Gold Standards Framework   www.goldstandardsframework.org.uk

Table 5.2 Advance Care Planning resources in the United Kingdom (continues opposite).

Advance care planning resources in the United Kingdon (continued)

Health and social care professional resources

Concise Guidance to Good Practice: No 12: Advance Care Planning
www.rcplondon.ac.uk/sites/default/files/documents/acp_web_final_21.01.09.pdf
Professional guide from the Royal College of Physicians

Capacity, Care Planning and Advance Care Planning in Life Limiting Illness: A Guide for Health and Social Care Staff
www.endoflifecareforadults.nhs.uk/assets/downloads/ACP_booklet_June_2011__with_links.pdf
Professional guide

Fact Sheet 2: Advance Care Planning
www.endoflifecareforadults.nhs.uk/publications/factsheet2
Overview for professionals

Advance Decisions to Refuse Treatment: A Guide for Health and Social Care Professionals
www.endoflifecareforadults.nhs.uk/publications/pubadrtguide
Professional guide

Fact Sheet 3: ADRT
www.endoflifecareforadults.nhs.uk/publications/factsheet3
Overview for professionals

The Differences Between General Care Planning and Decisions Made in Advance
www.endoflifecareforadults.nhs.uk/publications/differencesacpadrt
Chart clarifying the similarities and differences between general and ACP

Treatment and Care Towards the End of Life: Good Practice in Decision Making
www.gmc-uk.org/guidance/ethical_guidance/6858.asp
Professional guide including section on ACP

Planning Future Healthcare for People With Dementia Nearing End of Life
https://groups.its-services.org.uk/download/attachments/35686715/
Modernistation+Initiative_Planning+Future+Healthcare+for+end+of+life_Flowchart.pdf
Flow chart demonstrating necessary steps to take when discussing advance care planning with an individual with dementia

Table 5.2 Advance Care Planning resources in the United Kingdom (continued).

There are key communication, attitudes, behaviours and traits which facilitate communication, such as:

- empathy (the ability to understand an individual's feelings and demonstrate it);
- genuineness (the ability to be yourself despite your professional role); and
- respect (the ability to accept the patient as they are) [19].

Facilitative communication skills include: open questions (eg, *'How have things been?'*); open directive questions (eg, *'How have things been in the last few days?'*); questions with a psychological focus (eg, *'How have you been feeling about the last few days?'*); physical focus questions (eg, *'How has your breathlessness been in the last few days?'*); and questions that explore the psychological or physical focus (eg, 'You say that the breathlessness in the last few days has made you frightened?' or 'What frightens you when you got breathless?'). Empathy can help facilitate a conversation as well as enable the patient to feel validated in their experience (eg, 'I can see that the breathlessness is very worrying for you'). Screening questions help find out more information (eg, 'You mention the breathlessness; is there anything else to mention?'). Summarising helps to demonstrate empathy and that you have listened to the patient as well as confirm that you have the correct facts (eg, 'You have told me that you have been more breathless in the last few days and that this is more frightening for you').

There are a variety of models for breaking or communicating significant news which are helpful in communication on the subject of COPD (Table 5.3) [10].

Symptom control
Oxygen therapy

Although studies demonstrate a survival benefit for those using prolonged long-term oxygen therapy (LTOT) (>15 hours/day), no improvement in symptoms has been demonstrated. Equally, the use of oxygen on an as-needed basis is without definitive evidence to support it. However, small, but statistically significant ($P<0.05$) increases in taking a 6-minute walks using oxygen have been demonstrated. Overall, despite this lack of evidence, palliative oxygen for the management of breathlessness is commonly prescribed. This leads to its own problems in terms of treatment 'dependence' – patients may feel 'tied' to a machine, develop anxiety about the power supply and limit excursions outside the home. Abernethy et al reported on the effect of palliative oxygen versus room air for refractory dyspnoea, which revealed interesting results. They found that oxygen delivered by a nasal cannula provided no additional symptomatic benefit for relief of refractory dyspnoea in patients with life-limiting illness compared with room air, and that less burdensome strategies should be considered after brief assessment of the effect of oxygen therapy on the individual patient [20].

Opioids

Opioids (particularly morphine) have been used to treat refractory breathlessness for many years. However, there are safety concerns of respiratory depression and the perceived lack of evidence for their use [21]. In addition, there is also clinician reluctance to use opioids outside of the final days of life [22]. This makes it additionally challenging for the practitioner, considering the difficulty in prognostication or defining the end of life in COPD.

In 2001, Jennings et al conducted a systematic review of data on the use of opioids in COPD [23]. The analysis demonstrated a highly statistically significant effect of oral and parenteral opioids on the sensation of breathlessness (overall pooled effect size -0.31; 95% CI -0.50 to -0.13, $P=0.0008$). No significant adverse events were noted. Varkey examined the efficacy of opioids administered orally, in nebulised form and other routes, in dyspnoea relief and the factors that inhibit the prescription and use of opioids, and concluded that opioids are an effective palliative drug in patients with COPD and distressing dyspnoea refractory to standard modalities of treatment [24]. A review by Horton et al of opioid responsiveness in patients with COPD highlighted evidence of known dimensions that contribute to the sensation of dyspnoea in patients with COPD, building upon clinical observational experience to generate a conceptual model of opioid responsiveness [22]. They proposed a 'dyspnoea target' and 'opioid responsiveness score' as a means of more clearly defining the sensations encountered by a given patient and the likelihood of symptomatic improvement in response to opioids – an area for future research. Further evidence on the multidimensional aspects of dyspnoea will also provide more insights into the understanding of its role in COPD.

The alleviating effects of opioids on breathlessness can occur at low doses and persist for longer than expected. A 'start low and step up' approach is recommended, eg, a starting dose of 1.25–2.5 mg immediate-release morphine every 4 hours (with concurrent antiemetics and laxatives). Often the immediate-release morphine can be switched to a 12-hour long acting formulation once a stable regular dose has been

Models that can lend structure to Advance Care Planning discussions

SPIKES	PREPARED	SAGE & THYME	CALGARY-CAMBRIDGE
	Prepare for the discussion: Check patient's diagnosis and results; privacy; significant others **Relate to the person:** Develop rapport and show empathy	**Setting:** Create privacy and choose right time to discuss emotions and concerns	**Initiating the session:** Establish initial rapport; identify reason for consultation with open questions; listen without interrupting; confirm and screen for further problems; negotiate agenda
Perception: The 'before you tell, ask' principle; you should glean a fairly accurate picture of the patient's perception of their medical condition	**Elicit patient and caregiver preferences:** Clarify aim of meeting; elicit patient's understanding and expectations	**Ask:** Specific questions about feelings **Gather:** Make a list of things the patient tells you **Empathy:** See below **Talk:** Ask if patient has anyone they can talk to **Help:** Have they been helped in the past? **You:** 'What do you think would help?' **Me:** 'Would you like me to do anything?'	**Gathering information:** Explore patient's problems; open to closed questions; listen attentively; facilitate patient responses; pick up cues; clarify unclear statements; summarise periodically; use clear questions; establish a sequence of events; explore patient's ideas, concerns, expectations and feelings
Invitation: Check how much patient wants to know about diagnosis and treatment; obtaining overt permission respects the patient's right to know (or not to know)	**Provide information:** Offer to discuss issues, giving patient option not to discuss it		
			Providing structure: Summarise appropriately; signpost; use logical sequence; keep to time

Table 5.3 Models that can lend structure to Advance Care Planning discussions (continues opposite).

Models that can lend structure to Advance Care Planning discussions (continued)

SPIKES	PREPARED	SAGE & THYME	CALGARY-CAMBRIDGE
			Building relationship: Use appropriate non-verbal behaviour; develop rapport, use empathy, provide support; involve patient
Knowledge: Give information at patient's pace using the same language as them; 'chunk and check'	**Provide information:** Give information at patient's pace, using clear language; explain uncertainty; consider caregiver's and family's information needs		**Explanation and planning:** Correct amount and type of information; aid recall and understanding; shared understanding; shared decision-making
Empathy: Listen for, identify, acknowledge and validate emotions	**Acknowledge emotions and concerns:** Explore, acknowledge and respond to fears, concerns and emotions	**Empathy:** Use silence, give space, reflect patient's feelings	
	(Foster) Realistic hope: Be honest, offering appropriate reassurance but not false hope		
	Encourage questions and further discussions: Check understanding; emphasise discussion can be ongoing		
Strategy and summary: Summarise discussion, giving chance for questions or concerns; clarify next steps	**Document:** Write summary of discussion; contact other relevant practitioners	**End:** Reflect, acknowledge and conclude meeting, emphasizing main points	**Closing and planning:** Forward planning; summary; final check

Table 5.3 Models that can lend structure to Advance Care Planning discussions (continued). By permission of [10].

established. Opioids should be used only for the relief of dyspnoea, pain and sometimes cough. If and when sedation is needed, then judicious use of benzodiazepines may be considered.

Nebulised opioids

It is thought that nebulised opioids may act on a local level on peripheral receptors in small airways. Much like the data on oral opioids, the data for nebulised formulations are inconsistent across different advanced respiratory diseases. This approach is not routinely used.

Benzodiazepines

This group of drugs is sometimes used to relieve anxiety in the breathless patient, although caution should be used when considering them for patients with COPD. A review of 14 studies (200 patients with COPD and advanced cancer) found no evidence for a beneficial effect of benzodiazepines for the relief of breathlessness in this group of patients [25]. There was a slight but nonsignificant trend towards a beneficial effect, but the overall effect size was small. Benzodiazepines caused more drowsiness as an adverse effect than placebo, but less than morphine. These results justify considering benzodiazepines as a second- or third-line treatment within an individual therapeutic trial, when opioids and nonpharmacological measures have failed to control breathlessness [25]. Lorazepam 1–2 mg PRN and diazepam 2–5 mg BD or PRN can be helpful in emergency situations as well as diazepam 2–5 mg BD or PRN [26]. Occasionally, midazolam is also used and can be administered buccally as well as parentally [27].

Psychotropic drugs

The use of psychotropic agents in some individuals, including anxiolytics, phenothiazines and selective serotonin reuptake inhibitors, for the treatment of refractory dyspnoea has attracted some attention in the last few years due to the psychological component of refractory dyspnoea [28].

Emerging data

There has been a great deal of interest in treating refractory dyspnoea with therapies aimed at altering the perception of dyspnoea [29]. Investigators have looked at oral, nebulised, parenteral and inhaled opioids, psycho-tropic drugs, inhaled furosemide and heliox. Recent reports from Horton and Rocker [30] and Ora et al [31] found that current evidence supports further work in these areas. However, caution still needs to be applied. Inhaled furosemide has been studied in patients with COPD [32]. The rationale for its use is weak and based upon some properties as a cough suppressant and bronchodilator. On the other hand, furosemide may also act indirectly on vagally mediated sensory nerve endings in airway epithelium [33]. Studies have demonstrated a decrease in breathlessness as well as an increase in exercise capacity [36].

Heliox 28 is a helium/oxygen mixture containing 72% helium and 28% oxygen. This gas mixture has a low viscosity and so may decrease the work of breathing and thus reduce breathlessness. A recent multicentre, prospective, randomised, controlled trial carried out in seven intensive care units in Italy (N=204) showed only small trends favouring heliox [34]. Thus far, studies are inconclusive and the use of oxygen alone is probably as beneficial and more cost-effective.

TORCH (Towards a Revolution in COPD Health), a 3-year, multicentre, double-blind trial, enrolled >6100 patients with COPD into one of four treatment arms: salmeterol (50 μg) plus fluticasone propionate (500 μg) administered with a single inhaler; salmeterol alone (50 μg); fluticasone propionate alone (500 μg); or placebo [35]. The primary endpoint was all-cause mortality. Compared with placebo, the salmeterol/fluticasone combination reduced annual rates of COPD exacerbations and improved quality of life. However, the reduction in all-cause mortality among patients with COPD in the combination therapy group did not reach the predetermined level of statistical significance.

In a similar multicentre, double-blind trial, TRISTAN (Trial of Inhaled Steroids and long-acting β_2-agonists [LABAs]), 1465 patients with COPD were enrolled for a period of 1 year [36]. The primary endpoint was FEV_1 after 12 months' treatment and secondary endpoints included other lung function measurements, use of relief medication, respiratory symptoms, COPD exacerbations, health status and adverse events. There was a statistically significant benefit of the combination therapy over salmeterol alone in terms of FEV_1, but this only amounted to 48 mL on average and did not result in any significant benefit in health-related QOL. In this study, the LABAs alone reduced the exacerbation rate to a similar degree as the combination therapy or fluticasone alone.

In a study by Stoltz et al, 208 consecutive patients with COPD exacerbations were analysed. Measuring procalcitonin prior to commencement of antibiotic treatment gave clear indications as to which patients would benefit from treatment, with no long-term detriment to patient outcome (measured by FEV_1 at 14 days, rehospitalisation rate and time to next exacerbation). Antibiotic prescription was reduced from 72% to 40% ($P<0.0001$) [37].

Nonpharmacological interventions

The systematic review by Bausewein et al of nonpharmacological measures for the treatment of breathlessness in malignant and nonmalignant disease (including COPD) concluded that breathing training, walking aids, neuroelectrical muscle stimulation and chest wall vibration can all help breathlessness in advanced stages of disease [38].

Pulmonary rehabilitation

Pulmonary rehabilitation (PR) is a vital part of the care of patients with COPD and is recommended by all current COPD guidelines. Much of the patients' experience of COPD will happen in their home setting, so PR programmes can help them to feel empowered and independent. There is strong support for patients with COPD to initiate PR within one month following an acute exacerbation, as PR can provide improved dyspnoea, exercise tolerance and health-related QOL relative to usual care [39].

A meta-analysis of 31 randomised controlled trials investigated the effect of PR on health-related QOL and exercise capacity in patients with COPD [40]. In four important QOL domains (Chronic Respiratory Questionnaire scores for dyspnoea, fatigue, emotional function and mastery), the effect was larger than the minimal clinically important difference of 0.5 units. Statistically significant improvements were noted in two of the three domains of the St. George's Respiratory Questionnaire. Six-minute walking distance was improved, although slightly below threshold for clinical significance (weighted mean difference 48 m;

95% CI, 32–65; n=16 trials). This study reiterates the important and worthwhile objectives of PR [40].

Nutrition

Malnutrition is not uncommon in patients with COPD and weight loss can become particularly severe as the disease advances. Consequences of weight loss include muscular weakness leading to impaired lung function and breathlessness. Nutritional support is a simple, effective intervention in the management of patients with severe COPD.

Psychosocial support

Providing psychosocial support is a fundamental part of caring for any patient with chronic illness, but it becomes more important as patients begin to decline and experience increasing functional limitations. Patients and carers need help in coping with the illness and the changes occurring in their lives. Psychological support can include a variety of approaches in COPD, from advanced communication skills to cognitive behavioural therapy (CBT). Livermore et al [41] report the value of the CBT approach in panic attacks in COPD. Similarly, results from a randomised controlled trial of 25 patients indicated that CBT may provide rapid symptom relief for patients with COPD and clinically significant anxiety and depression [42].

Breathing techniques

Several controlled breathing techniques, including positioning and pursed lip breathing, may be useful in the management of breathlessness. For example, pursed lip breathing has been shown to decrease air trapping by increasing positive end-expiratory pressure and preventing dynamic airway collapse. Findings from a recent study also support the idea that a handheld fan directed to the face reduces the sensation of breathlessness and may be recommended as part of a management strategy for treating breathlessness associated with advanced disease [43].

Breathlessness clinics

For some time now, 'breathlessness clinics' have been run by nurse practitioners and physiotherapists, although they primarily serve patients with lung cancer [27]. Hately et al [45] reported highly significant improvements in breathlessness, functional capacity, activity levels and distress levels in patients with lung cancer who had visited a breathlessness clinic. The percentage of patients experiencing breathlessness several times or more per day was reduced from 73% to 27% four weeks later While similar studies have not been conducted in patients with COPD, they could potentially derive the same benefit [27].

The future of palliative care in COPD

As individuals continue to live longer, the number of patients with end-stage COPD patients will increase. Palliative interventions for those with advanced COPD have the potential to reduce the suffering caused by this progressive disease. Coordinating, planning and delivering care across the settings will need to be carefully coordinated with established palliative and respiratory care services. Recognising the physical, emotional, psychological, social and spiritual needs of this group of patients will aid this planning and delivery of services. There need to be additional studies about the experience of living with COPD, the mechanisms of dyspnoea and symptom control management plans. The ACP process and the communication skills that are part of that process will need to be facilitated by a confident and competent workforce in order to increase the possibility of patients living and dying in their preferred place of care and death.

References

1 Seamark DA, Seamark CJ, Halpin DM. Palliative care in chronic obstructive pulmonary disease: a review for clinicians. J R Soc Med 2007; 100:225–233.

2 World Health Organization. National Cancer Control Programmes: Policies and Managerial Guidelines. 2002. Available at: http://whqlibdoc.who.int/hq/2002/9241545577.pdf. Last accessed October 2012.

3 Roberts CM, Seiger A, Buckingham RJ, Stone RA. Clinician perceived good practice in end-of-life care for patients with COPD. Palliat Med 2008; 22:855–858.

4 Department of Health. End of Life Care Strategy Promoting High Quality Care for All Adults at the End of Life. 2008. Available at: www.dh.gov.uk/prod_consum_dh/groups/ dh_digitalassets/@dh/@en/documents/digitalasset/dh_086345.pdf. Last accessed October 2012.

5 Skilbeck J, Mott L, Page H, et al. Palliative care in chronic obstructive airways disease: a needs assessment. Palliat Med 1998; 12:245–254.

6 Gore JM, Brophy CJ, Greenstone MA. How well do we care for patients with end stage chronic obstructive pulmonary disease (COPD)? A comparison of palliative care and quality of life in COPD and lung cancer. Thorax 2000; 55:1000–1006.

7 Lokke A, Lange P, Scharling H, et al. Developing COPD: a 25 year follow up study of the general population. Thorax 2006; 61:935–939.

8 National Health Service. Capacity, Care Planning and Advance Care Planning in Life Limiting Illness: A Guide for Health and Social Care Staff. Available at: www.endoflifecareforadults. nhs.uk/assets/downloads/ACP_booklet_June_2011__with_links.pdf. Last accessed October 2012.

9 Royal College of Physicians. Concise Guidance to Good Practice: No 12: Advance Care Planning 2009. London, UK; Royal College of Physicians, 2009.

10 Bevan J, Fowler C, Russell S. Communication skills and advance care planning. In: Thomas K, Lobo B, eds. Advance Care Planning in End of Life Care. Oxford, UK: Oxford University Press, 2010; 261-276.

11 Gott M, Gardiner C, Small N, et al. Barriers to advance care planning in chronic obstructive pulmonary disease. Palliat Med 2009; 23:642–648.

12 Jones I, Kirby A, Ormiston P, et al. The needs of patients dying of chronic obstructive pulmonary disease in the community. Fam Pract 2004; 21:310–313.

13 Schwartz C. Decision making at the end of life: shifting sands. J R Soc Med 2005; 98:297–298.

14 Couceiro Vidal A, Pandiella A. COPD. A model for using advanced directives and care planning. Arch Bronconeumol 2010; 46:325–331.

15 Glaser BG, Strauss AL. Time for Dying. Chicago, IL: Aldine-Atherton, 1968.

16 Murray SA, Boyd K, Sheikh A. Palliative care in chronic illness. BMJ 2005; 330:611–612.

17 Curtis JR, Engelberg RA, Nielsen EL, et al. Patient-physician communication about end-of-life care for patients with severe COPD. Eur Respir J 2004; 24:200–205.

18 Curtis JR. Palliative and end-of-life care for patients with severe COPD. Eur Respir J 2008; 32:796–803.

19 Coulehan JL, Block MR. The Medical Interview: Mastering Skills for Clinical Practice, 5th Edition. Philadelphia, PA: F.A. Davis Co. School of Medicine, 2006.

20 Abernethy AP, McDonald CF, Frith PA, et al. Effect of palliative oxygen versus room air in relief of breathlessness in patients with refractory dyspnoea: a double-blind, randomised controlled trial. Lancet 2010; 376:784–793.

21 Pauwels RA, Buist AS, Calverley PM, et al. Global Strategy for the Diagnosis, Management, and Prevention of Chronic Obstructive Pulmonary Disease NHLBI/WHO Global Initiative for Chronic Obstructive Lung Disease (GOLD) Workshop Summary. Am J Respir Crit Care Med 2001; 163:1256–1276.

22 Horton R, Rocker G, Currow D. The dyspnea target: can we zero in on opioid responsiveness in advanced chronic obstructive pulmonary disease? Curr Opin Support Palliat Care 2010; 4:92–96.

23 Jennings AL, Davies AN, Higgins JP, et al. A systematic review of the use of opioids in the management of dyspnoea. Thorax 2002; 57:939–944.

24 Varkey B. Opioids for palliation of refractory dyspnea in chronic obstructive pulmonary disease patients. Curr Opin Pulm Med 2010; 16:150–154.

25 Simon ST, Higginson IJ, Booth S, et al. Benzodiazepines for the relief of breathlessness in advanced malignant and non-malignant diseases in adults. Cochrane Database Syst Rev 2010; 20:CD007354.

26 Watson M, Lucas C, Hoy A. Adult Palliative Care Guidance. 2nd ed. South West London, Surrey, West Sussex and Hampshire, Mount Vernon and Sussex Cancer Networks and Northern Ireland Palliative Medicine Group, 2006. Available at: www.communityhospice. org.uk/media/clinical%20guidelines.pdf. Last accessed October 2012.

27 Uronis HE, Currow DC, Abernethy A. Palliative management of refractory dyspnea in COPD. Int J Chron Obstruct Pulmon Dis 2006; 1:289–304.

28 Dean M. End of life care for COPD patients. Prim Care Resp J 2010; 17:46–50.

29 Burdon JG, Pain MC, Rubinfeld AR, et al. Chronic lung diseases and the perception of breathlessness: a clinical perspective. Eur Respir J 1994; 7:1342–1349.

30 Horton R, Rocker G. Contemporary issues in refractory dyspnoea in advanced chronic obstructive pulmonary disease. Curr Opin Support Palliat Care 2010; 4:56–62.

31 Ora J, Jensen D, O'Donnell DE. Exertional dyspnea in chronic obstructive pulmonary disease: mechanisms and treatment approaches. Curr Opin Pulm Med 2010; 16:144–149.

32 Ong KC, Kor AC, Chong WF, et al. Effects of inhaled furosemide on exertional dyspnea in chronic obstructive pulmonary disease. Am J Respir Crit Care Med 2004; 169:1028–1033.

33 Chung KF, Barnes PJ. Loop diuretics and asthma. Pulm Pharmacol 1992; 5:1–7.

34 Maggiore SM, Richard JC, Abroug F, et al. A multicenter, randomized trial of noninvasive ventilation with helium-oxygen mixture in exacerbations of chronic obstructive lung disease. Crit Care Med 2010; 38:145–151.

35 Calverly PM, Anderson JA, Celli B, et al.; TORCH investigators. Salmeterol and fluticasone propionate and survival in chronic obstructive pulmonary disease. N Engl J Med 2007; 356:775–789.

36 Calverley P, Pauwels R, Vestbo J, et al.; TRial of Inhaled STeroids ANd long-acting beta2 agonists study group. Combined salmeterol and fluticasone in the treatment of chronic obstructive pulmonary disease: a randomised controlled trial. Lancet 2003; 361:449–456.

37 Stolz D, Christ-Crain M, Bingisser R, et al. Antibiotic treatment of exacerbations of COPD: a randomized, controlled trial comparing procalcitonin-guidance with standard therapy. Chest 2007; 131:9–19.

38 Bausewein C, Booth S, Gysels M, Higginson I. Non-pharmacological interventions for breathlessness in advanced stages of malignant and non-malignant diseases. Cochrane Database Syst Rev 2008; 16:CD005623.

39 Marciniuk D, Brooks D, Butcher S, et al.; The Canadian Thoracic Society COPD Committee Expert Working Group. Optimizing pulmonary rehabilitation in chronic obstructive pulmonary disease – practical issues: A Canadian Thoracic Society Clinical Practice Guideline. Can Respir J 2010; 17:159–168.

40 Lacasse Y, Goldstein R, Lasserson TJ, et al. Pulmonary rehabilitation for chronic obstructive pulmonary disease. Cochrane Database Syst Rev 2006; :CD003793.

41 Livermore N, Sharpe L, McKenzie D. Panic attacks and panic disorder in chronic obstructive pulmonary disease: a cognitive behavioral perspective. Respir Med 2010; 104:1246–1253.

42 Hynninen MJ, Bjerke N, Pallesen S, et al. A randomized controlled trial of cognitive behavioral therapy for anxiety and depression in COPD. Respir Med 2010; 104:986–994.

43 Galbraith S, Fagan P, Perkins P, et al. Does the use of a handheld fan improve chronic dyspnea? A randomized, controlled, crossover trial. J Pain Symptom Manage 2010; 39:831–838.

44 Hately J, Laurence V, Scott A, et al. Breathlessness clinics within specialist palliative care settings can improve the quality of life and functional capacity of patients with lung cancer. Palliat Med 2003; 17:410–417.

Chapter 6

The future of COPD

The past 10 years have seen major changes in the way we look at chronic obstructive pulmonary disease and how we manage it. At present, we still have yet to find a therapy that changes the prognosis or reverses disease progression [1], with smoking cessation being the only effective intervention to achieve this.

New bronchodilators

Bronchodilators are currently the main treatment used for the relief of breathlessness in COPD, but they do not directly affect the underlying disease process even though they are effective at reducing exacerbation rates. Long-acting bronchodilators are the preferred therapy, including the anticholinergic (anti-muscarinic) tiotropium bromide and the long-acting β_2-agonists (LABAs) salmeterol and formoterol. Importantly, there is an additive effect between tiotropium and formoterol (Figure 6.1) [2]. Thus, possibilities exist for the development of fixed-combination inhalers containing both a long-acting anticholinergic and a LABA, particularly an ultra-LABA (uLABA). This emerging combination modality is now an area of fierce competition.

The long-acting muscarinic antagonist (LAMA) aclidinium bromide **was approved in the United States and Europe in July 2012 [3,4].** Glycopyrronium bromide was approved in Europe in October 2012 and an application is expected to be filed in the United States in 2014. Several other LAMAs with an action of over 24 hours are now in development, including glycopyrrolate and LAS34273 (Table 6.1) [5,6]. Currently

R. E. K. Russell et al., *Managing COPD*,
DOI: 10.1007/978-1-907673-52-8_6, © Springer Healthcare 2013

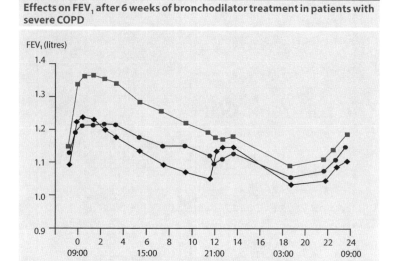

Figure 6.1 Effects on FEV₁ after 6 weeks of bronchodilator treatment in patients with severe COPD. Mean FEV₁ (adjusted for period, centre and patient within centre) before and during 24 hours after the inhalation of tiotropium once daily (●), formoterol twice daily (◆) and tiotropium plus formoterol once daily (■) at the end of the 6-week treatment period. Reproduced with permission from [2].

available LABAs need to be given twice a day, and so are not ideal for the fixed LABA/LAMA combination. Table 6.2 lists novel LABA/LAMA combinations in development [5,7]. The uLABA indacaterol was approved in Europe in 2009 and in the United States in 2011 [8,9]. Some uLABAs in development are listed in Table 6.3 [5,7,10]. Theoretically, LABA/corticosteroid combination inhalers should be more effective than LABAs or corticosteroids alone owing to increased glucocorticoid receptor translocation. This has been reflected in data from the Towards a Revolution in COPD Health (TORCH) study [11]. Primary endpoint all-cause mortality rates were 12.6% in the combination therapy group, 15.2% in the placebo group, 13.5% in the salmeterol group and 16.0% in the fluticasone group, although the difference did not reach clinical significance. In the future, it should be feasible to put all three medications together (uLABA, LAMA and a once-daily steroid). This could further enhance any potential additive effects of these drugs.

Novel LAMAs undergoing development			
Drug	Advantages	Latest developments	Company working on this strategy
Umeclidinium bromide	Long duration of action when administered via inhalation in animal models supports the potential for use as a once-daily bronchodilator for COPD. Clinical data have not been disclosed	Phase III	GlaxoSmithKline, London, UK
TD-4208	Significant improvement in lung function versus placebo; comparable to ipratropium bromide. Rapid mechanism of action. Well tolerated; most common side effects are headache and dyspnoea	Phase IIa	Theravance, South San Francisco, CA, USA
CHF 5407	An antagonist as potent and long-acting as tiotropium on human M_3 muscarinic receptors, but significantly short-acting on M_2 receptors. Duration of action is similar to that of tiotropium	Phase I/II	Chiesi Farmaceutici, Parma, Italy

Table 6.1 Novel LAMAs undergoing development. LAMAs, long-acting anti-muscarinic antagonists; ACCLAIM: AClidinium CLinical Trial Assessing Efficacy and Safety In Moderate to Severe COPD Patients. Data adapted from [5,6].

More effective smoking cessation

Smoking cessation is a vital part of COPD management. Clinicians should be prepared to intervene in cases where patients are willing to quit; supportive strategies such as the 'five As' (ask, advise, assess, assist, arrange) can be beneficial (see Table 6.4) [12]. However, current smoking cessation strategies, including behavioural approaches, hypnosis and nicotine replacement therapy (NRT), have very low success rates, although recently it has become clear that prior use of NRT before smoking cessation can improve quit rates. One of the most effective pharmacological agents available is bupropion, but in patients with COPD the annual quit rate is only 15%. This indicates that more effective smoking cessation therapies are needed in the future. Several new classes of non-nicotinic drugs for smoking cessation are now in development (see Table 6.5). Varenicline, a partial nicotine agonist which targets the $\alpha_4\beta_2$-nicotinic acetylcholine receptor, was licensed in 2006. Despite carrying a black-box

Novel combinations of LABAs and LAMAs undergoing development

Drug(s)	Advantages	Latest developments	Company working on this strategy
Vilaterol/ umeclidinium bromide	Statistically significant improvements in lung function vs. placebo, vilaterol alone, and tiotropium. Few serious side effects	Phase III	GlaxoSmithKline, London, UK/ Theravance, South San Francisco, CA, USA
Indacaterol/ glycopyrronium bromide (QVA-149)	Superior effect on lung outcome and functions	Phase III	Novartis, Basel, Switzerland
Aclidinium/ formoterol (LAS40464)	No data presented yet. It should be established whether formoterol can be administered on a once-daily basis	Phase III	Almirall Prodesfarma, Barcelona, Spain
Olodaterol/ tiotropium	Significant improvements in lung function over 24 hours versus olodaterol alone. Safe and well tolerated. Current Phase III program (TOviTO) underway	Phase II/III	Boehringer Ingelheim, Ingelheim, Germany
Glycopyrrolate/ formoterol (PT003)	Significant improvement in peak expiratory flow rates compared with its individual components and tiotropium. Reduced albuterol usage. Safe and well tolerated.	Phase IIb	Pearl Therapeutics, Redwood City, CA, USA
GSK-961081	It is both a muscarinic antagonist and a β_2-adrenoceptor agonist. It is at least equivalent to 50 µg salmeterol b.i.d. plus 18 µg tiotropium q.d.	Phase II	GlaxoSmithKline, London, UK/Theravance, South San Francisco, CA, USA
Carmoterol/ tiotropium	No data presented yet	Phase I/II	Chiesi Farmaceutici, Parma, Italy
Formoterol/ dexpirronium	No data presented yet. It should be established whether formoterol can be administered on a once-daily basis	Phase I	Meda Pharmaceuticals, Solna, Sweden

Table 6.2 Novel combinations of LABAs and LAMAs undergoing development. LABAs, long-acting β_2-agonists; LAMA, long-acting anti-muscarinic antagonists. Data adapted from [5,7].

drug warning when the long-term results of two licensing studies were pooled (Table 6.6), varenicline more than doubled the odds of stopping smoking compared with placebo (odds ratio [OR] 2.82; 95% confidence interval [CI] 2.06–3.86) and was significantly better than bupropion (OR 1.56; 95% CI 1.19–2.06) [13,14].

Another approach that may have longer term benefits is the development of a vaccine against nicotine, which stimulates the production of antibodies that bind nicotine so that it cannot enter the brain. However,

uLABAs undergoing development

Drug	Advantages	Latest developments	Company working on this strategy
Carmoterol	Binds very firmly to the β_2-adrenoceptor. Highly potent and selective. Displays fast onset and long duration of activity in both asthma and COPD at very low dosage (2–4 µg)	Launch aimed for late 2013	Chiesi Farmaceutici, Parma, Italy
Vilanterol	Potent, selective β_2-adrenoceptor agonist. Displays a long duration of activity in both asthma and COPD. Safe and well tolerated, with the most frequently reported adverse event being headache.	No plans for single launch — will concentrate on combinations	GlaxoSmithKline, London, UK/Theravance, San Francisco, CA, USA
Olodaterol	Potent β_2-adrenoceptor agonist. Seems to be equivalent to formoterol for speed of onset and efficacy, but with a longer duration of action. Displays a long duration of activity (24-h) in both asthma and COPD	Phase II/III	Boehringer Ingelheim, Ingelheim, Germany
Abediterol	24-h duration of activity in asthma	No plans for single launch — will concentrate on combinations with inhaled corticosteroids	Almirall Prodesfarma, Barcelona, Spain

Table 6.3 uLABAs undergoing development. uLABAs, ultra-long-acting β_2-agonists. Data adapted from [5,7,10].

the first nicotine vaccine to make it to that stage failed two large Phase III trials, as efficacy was found to be no different from placebo. It is unclear as to whether further development will continue.

The problem of corticosteroid resistance in COPD

In sharp contrast to patients with asthma, patients with COPD show a poor response to inhaled corticosteroids, suggesting that there is a degree of resistance to their anti-inflammatory effects. There may be several reasons for corticosteroid resistance in COPD; one of the most convincing is a reduction in the nuclear enzyme histone deacetylase 2 (HDAC2), which is recruited by the activated glucocorticoid receptor to switch off inflammatory gene transcription. There is a marked reduction

The 'five As' strategy for patients willing to quit tobacco use	
Ask	Systematically identify all tobacco users at every visit
	Implement a system that ensures that for every patient at every clinic visit, tobacco use status is queried and documented
Advise	In a clear, strong and personalised manner, urge every tobacco user to quit
Assess	Determine willingness to make a quit attempt
	Ask every tobacco user if he or she is willing to make a quit attempt at this time (ie, within the next 30 days)
Assist	Aid the patient with a quit plan
	Provide practical counselling
	Provide intra-treatment social support
	Help the patient obtain extra-treatment social support
	Recommend use of approved pharmacotherapy except in special circumstances
	Provide supplementary materials
Arrange	Schedule follow-up contact, either in person or via telephone

Table 6.4 The 'five As' strategy for patients willing to quit tobacco use. Adapted from [12].

Drugs for smoking cessation
Current therapies
Nicotine replacement
Bupropion
Varenicline
Future therapies
Gamma-aminobutyric acid B agonists
Nicotine vaccine

Table 6.5 Drugs for smoking cessation.

in HDAC2 activity in the peripheral lung, preventing corticosteroids from switching off inflammation [15]. This reduction in HDAC2 appears to be the result of oxidative and nitrative stress, both of which are increased in patients with COPD. This provides an alternative strategy for the development of new treatments. Theoretically, antioxidants should reverse corticosteroid resistance, but current drugs are not efficient. Inhibitors of nitric oxide generation should also be effective, and several potent inhibitors of inducible nitric oxide synthase are now in clinical development. Unexpectedly, low-dose theophylline seems to act as a novel HDAC activator and is able to reverse corticosteroid resistance in both animal models of smoking and cells taken from humans with COPD [16]. Two recent studies [17,18] have explored whether theophylline can

Cessation rates of two randomised controlled outcome trials				
	End of treatment		One-year follow-up	
	Study 1	Study 2	Study 1	Study 2
Varenicline	44	44	22	23
Bupropion	30	30	16	15
Placebo	18	18	8	10

Table 6.6 Cessation rates of two randomised controlled outcome trials. Treatment is for 12 weeks. Numbers in table are % abstinent (weeks 9–12 in 'end of treatment'). Conventional rounding was used: 0.1–0.4, rounded down; 0.5–0.9, rounded up. Data from [13,14].

reverse steroid resistance in patients wth COPD. It is hopeful that this will lead to the development of a large clinical trial to determine whether disease progression can be halted. This would revolutionise the management of COPD. Furthermore, theophylline is inexpensive and raises no safety concerns when the low doses ($\sim$5–10 mg/L) required to increase HDAC levels are used.

New treatments for COPD

New therapies are desperately needed for COPD, particularly anti-inflammatory therapies to prevent exacerbations and disease progression [19]. Testing drugs in COPD is a major challenge. High dropout rates make it difficult to devise long-term large studies. However, proof-of-concept clinical studies are more easily performed. There is some research interest in the molecular and cell biology of COPD in order to identify novel therapeutic targets. Animal models of COPD for early drug testing are poor and focus on emphysema, rather than the small airway disease that appears to underlie the progressive loss of FEV_1 and the increasing symptoms over time that are characteristic of COPD. Better animal models that have predominantly small airway disease are urgently needed.

There are also uncertainties about how to test drugs for COPD, which may require long-term studies (over 1 year) in relatively large numbers of patients at an enormous cost. For example, the TORCH trial, which looked at the effects of drug intervention on mortality, cost several hundred million dollars. Furthermore, many patients with COPD will have comorbidities such as ischaemic heart disease and diabetes, which may exclude them from clinical trials of new therapies. There is little information about how surrogate markers like biomarkers in the blood, sputum or breath, may help to monitor the short-term efficacy and predict the long-term potential of new treatments. Finally, it is difficult to accurately measure small airway function in patients with COPD, so there is a need to develop better tests of small airway function that are not affected by emphysema or abnormalities of large airway function [20].

Several new classes of anti-inflammatory drugs are now in clinical development for COPD. The most advanced of these new drugs are phosphodiesterase (PDE)4 inhibitors, which increase cyclic adenosine monophosphate concentrations in inflammatory cells and have a broad spectrum of anti-inflammatory effects (Figure 6.2) [21–23]. The dose has been limited by side effects, particularly nausea and gastrointestinal problems. In 2011, roflumilast was approved by the FDA as an add-on treatment to reduce the risk of COPD exacerbations in patients with severe COPD associated with chronic bronchitis and a history of exacerbations [24]. More selective inhibitors (PDE4B inhibitors) and administration through inhalation (although this too has proved disappointing) are currently being investigated to try and limit side effects.

Several other broad-spectrum anti-inflammatory therapies are currently under investigation (Figure 6.2), but most of these are likely to have side effects when given systemically, so inhaled administration may be required.

Mediator antagonists

Many mediators are now implicated in COPD, including lipid mediators and cytokines [25]. Although inhibiting specific mediators, by receptor antagonists or synthesis inhibitors, is a relatively easy approach, this is unlikely to produce very effective drugs owing to the large amount of redundancy within these biological systems, an example of which is the failure of p38 blockade in rheumatoid arthritis (although this may be a useful therapy in acute exacerbations of COPD). The premise of mediator blockade is to 'take out' the insulting raised cytokine/chemokine (Figure 6.3) [23]. This can be achieved by small molecule inhibition (low molecular weight) or biological targeting through receptor or moiety antibody blockade (high molecular weight or so-called 'biologics').

Potential targets in COPD: role of anti-inflammatory drugs

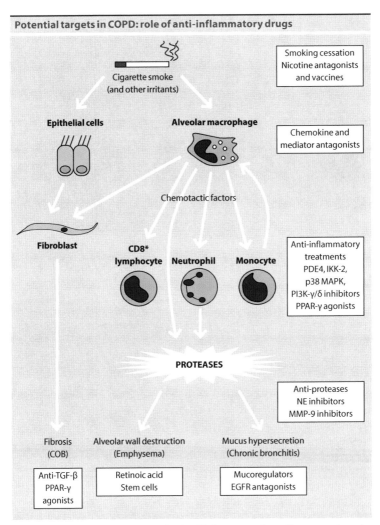

Figure 6.2 Potential targets in COPD: role of anti-inflammatory drugs. Cigarette smoke and other irritants activate macrophages in the respiratory tract that release multiple chemotactic factors that attract neutrophils, monocytes and T-lymphocytes (particularly CD8* cells). Several cells also release proteases, such as neutrophil elastase (NE) and matrix metalloproteinase-9 (MMP-9), which break down connective tissue in the lung parenchyma (emphysema) and also stimulate mucus hypersecretion (chronic bronchitis). CD8* may also be involved in alveolar wall destruction. This inflammatory process may be inhibited at several stages (shown in boxes). PDE, phosphodiesterase; IKK, inhibitor of nuclear factor-κB kinase; MAPK, mitogen-activated protein kinase; PI3K, phosphoinositide-3-kinase; PPAR, peroxisome proliferator activated receptor; COB, chronic obstructive bronchitis; TGF, transforming growth factor; CB, cannabinoid; EGFR, epithelial growth factor receptor. Reproduced with permission from [23].

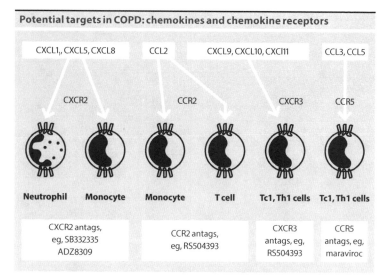

Figure 6.3 Potential targets in COPD: chemokines and chemokine receptors. Several chemokines and chemokine receptors are involved in the inflammation of COPD. Chemokines released from epithelial cells and macrophages in the lung recruit inflammatory cells (Tc1 CD8* T lymphocytes, neutrophils and monocytes) from the circulation. Small molecule chemokine receptor agtagonists are now in development (shown in boxes). Reproduced with permission from [23].

Further engineering of these molecules can improve efficacy, eg, the development of nanobodies and diabodies. Anti-TNF antibodies are currently used to treat patients with severe rheumatoid arthritis and inflammatory bowel disease, but so far these appear to be disappointing in COPD. An IL-8-blocking antibody has also proved to be largely ineffective in COPD. Although other biological targets are being pursued, it remains to be seen whether the efficacy of these products can be measured in an acceptable timeframe.

Protease inhibitors

Several proteases, particularly elastases, have been implicated in alveolar destruction, and are a target for therapy in patients with COPD and emphysema. Proteases may be inhibited by administering their endogenous antiproteases, such as α_1-antitrypsin, or small molecule inhibitors. So far, no clinical studies have demonstrated that these approaches have any effect in COPD.

Lung repair

COPD is largely irreversible, but it is possible that efforts to enhance the remodelling process may restore lung function. There has been particular interest in retinoic acid, which is able to reverse experimental emphysema in rats; however, this is unlikely to work in humans, whose lungs do not have the same regenerative capacity. There are now small mediators that have been specifically implicated in restorative functions, eg, resolvins, and these may be of interest in the future. Another novel approach that is being actively explored is the use of stem cells (distil airway stem cells expressing p63/Krt5) to regenerate epithelial/alveolar cells within the lung, though the possibility of unchecked cellular division could lead to an unacceptable increase in solid tumour growth.

Biomarkers of COPD

Predicting disease susceptibility to the effects of cigarette smoke is perhaps the most important potential use of any biomarker in COPD. Efforts in this area in particular genetic analysis of single nucleotide polymorphisms using gene-chip technology, have yet to make a breakthrough. Whilst the search continues for useful disease indicators, the use of pro-calcitonin in the prognostication of exacerbation severity has shown some promise. Tools are being developed which help predict exacerbations, such as the EXACT-PRO model advocated by the FDA and the DOSE Index [26,27]. Ultimately, these may be made available to patients via PDA (personal digital assistant) platforms. Sensitive measures of small airway function are now being more widely used, such as X5 (reactance) using impulse oscillometry and the older technique of multiple breath nitrogen washout. New imaging techniques, such as MRI scanning with radiolabelled helium and xenon, also offer promise as they do not involve large amounts of ionising radiation, a problem with high-resolution computed tomography. The use of the apparent diffusion coefficient within this context shows promise. Utilizing autofluoresence to directly image cells within the alveoli/terminal airways also has a great deal of potential [28]. Induced sputum is still employed in many proof-of-concept trials. It is now widely accepted that sputum neutrophils and IL-8 are good valid measures of airway inflammation if used correctly.

Routes of drug delivery

Traditionally, drugs for airway diseases are given by inhalation, but inhaler devices usually target larger airways, such as those implicated in asthma. In COPD, the inflammation is mainly in the smaller airways and the lung parenchyma, suggesting that inhalers which deliver drugs more peripherally may be more useful. Small particle inhalers, such as hydrofluoroalkane–beclomethasone propionate, used for asthma control, may be attractive in COPD because the inhaled drug would reach the lung periphery. Small volume nebulisers, eg, Respimat® Soft Mist™ inhaler, may also prove more effective, through low flow and a reduced particle size via a 'mist' formulation. Recent studies comparing the Handihaler and Respimat inhalers showed equivalent efficacy, measured by trough FEV_1 (5 μg Respimat SMI tiotropium versus 18 μg HandiHaler [29,30]). Oral therapy may treat systemic complications such as muscle wasting, weight loss and osteoporosis, which are a problem in patients with severe disease, although this carries an increased risk of side effects. Another experimental approach could exploit specific cell uptake mechanisms in target cells, such as macrophages.

Nonpharmacological treatments

Several nonpharmacological treatments are increasingly used as a complement to drug therapy. Nutritional supplements may have some benefit, but most research has focused on pulmonary rehabilitation (PR). This has been shown to improve exercise performance and health status in patients with COPD [31]. Pulmonary rehabilitation also reduces the utilisation of healthcare resources. Future PR programmes are likely to be community-based and consist of highly focused interactive sessions. Ongoing care taking place after the initial PR programme, including telephone calls, could be beneficial and may improve the long-term outcome, although this has not been studied systematically. An important area of development is the positive interaction between PR and current pharmacological therapies, particularly bronchodilators. Also, non-invasive ventilation in patients with severe ventilatory limitation appears to enhance the effects of exercise training.

In the future, better predictors of response are required, together with strategies that combine PR with other therapies such as treatments to enhance muscle strength. Unfortunately, one of the major barriers to the implementation of PR is the availability of trained staff. An organised integrated PR programme should be available to all patients seen at any tertiary referral unit.

Integrated care

It is now apparent that COPD is a highly complex disease with several systemic manifestations as well as associations with severe comorbidities, particularly cardiovascular disease. This means that a multidisciplinary approach is needed, with the participation of respiratory specialists, GPs, specialist nurses, physiotherapists and others (Figure 6.4) [32]. There will be a trend towards evaluating not only airflow limitation, but also systemic effects and comorbidities to optimise QOL.

COPD in the developing world

As Western governments impose smoking bans and legislate against smoking advertising, tobacco companies are increasingly turning their attention to the developing world. Higher levels of cigarette smoking correlates well with greater prosperity. Thus, not only will the burden of COPD increase but also the prevalence of other smoking-related diseases, leading to more premature deaths. For example, Central and Eastern Europe have the highest lung cancer rates in the world for men [33]. Low birth weight and the burning of biomass fuels also amplify the risks of cigarette smoke exposure. Emerging economies need the support of the developed world in order to prevent a forthcoming epidemic of COPD and smoking-related diseases. The developed world must set the agenda for change and lead by example. The countries of Eastern Europe, India and China are at risk of repeating all of the mistakes made in Western Europe and the United States in the 1960s and 1970s.

Conclusions

Over the next 10 years, there are likely to be various developments that will improve the management of COPD. Combination long-acting bronchodilators are the treatment of choice for symptom relief and reduce exacerbation rates, but there is a pressing need for effective anti-inflammatory

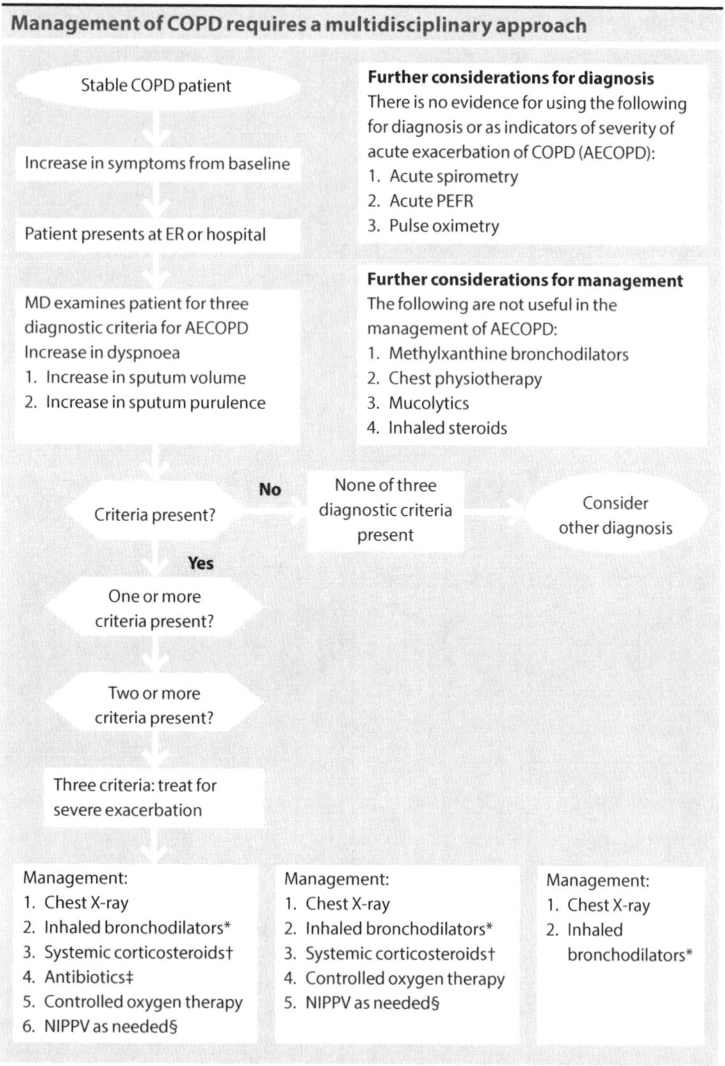

Management of COPD requires a multidisciplinary approach

Stable COPD patient

↓

Increase in symptoms from baseline

↓

Patient presents at ER or hospital

↓

MD examines patient for three diagnostic criteria for AECOPD
Increase in dyspnoea
1. Increase in sputum volume
2. Increase in sputum purulence

↓

Criteria present? — **No** → None of three diagnostic criteria present → Consider other diagnosis

Yes

↓

One or more criteria present?

↓

Two or more criteria present?

↓

Three criteria: treat for severe exacerbation

Further considerations for diagnosis
There is no evidence for using the following for diagnosis or as indicators of severity of acute exacerbation of COPD (AECOPD):
1. Acute spirometry
2. Acute PEFR
3. Pulse oximetry

Further considerations for management
The following are not useful in the management of AECOPD:
1. Methylxanthine bronchodilators
2. Chest physiotherapy
3. Mucolytics
4. Inhaled steroids

Management:
1. Chest X-ray
2. Inhaled bronchodilators*
3. Systemic corticosteroids†
4. Antibiotics‡
5. Controlled oxygen therapy
6. NIPPV as needed§

Management:
1. Chest X-ray
2. Inhaled bronchodilators*
3. Systemic corticosteroids†
4. Controlled oxygen therapy
5. NIPPV as needed§

Management:
1. Chest X-ray
2. Inhaled bronchodilators*

Figure 6.4 Management of COPD requires a multidisciplinary approach. *Use anticholinergic bronchodilators first, once at maximum dose, then add β_2-agonist bronchodilators. †Dosing regimen used in the SCOPE trial: 3 days intravenous methylprednisolone, 125 mg every 6 hours followed by oral prednisolone, taper to complete the 2-week course (60 mg/day on days 4–7, 40 mg/day on days 8–11, and 20 mg/day on days 12–15). ‡Use narrow-spectrum antibiotics: the agents favoured in the trials were amoxicillin, trimethoprim–sulphamethoxazole and tetracycline. §Non-invasive positive pressure ventilation should be administered under the surpervision of a trained physician. There are multiple components of COPD that need to be taken account in the management of this complex disease. This requires integrated care and a multidisciplinary approach. ER, emergency room; NIPPV, noninvasive positive pressure ventilation; PEFR, peak expiratory flow rate; URTI, upper respiratory tract infection. Adapted from [32].

treatments, particularly in patients who have ceased smoking. It is hoped that this will prevent disease progression. Various biomarkers are being developed to monitor pulmonary inflammation in COPD. Pulmonary rehabilitation is now well established and could be delivered more in the community in the future. In short, COPD is a multidimensional disease that requires an integrated multidisciplinary approach.

References

1   Barnes PJ, Stockley RA. COPD: current therapeutic interventions and future approaches. Eur Respir J 2005; 25:1084–1106.

2   van Noord JA, Aumann JL, Janssens E, et al. Comparison of tiotropium once daily, formoterol twice daily and both combined once daily in patients with COPD. Eur Respir J 2005; 26:214–222.

3   Tudorza Pressair [package insert]. St. Louis, MO: Forest Pharmaceuticals, Inc.; 2012.

4   European Medicines Agency. Summary of product characteristics for Eklira Genuair. Available at: www.ema.europa.eu/docs/en_GB/document_library/EPAR_-_Product_Information/human/002211/WC500132661.pdf. Last accessed October 2012.

5   Cazzola M, Matera MG. Emerging inhaled bronchodilators: an update. Eur Respir J 2009; 34:757-769.

6   Villetti G, Pastore F, Bergamaschi M, et al. Bronchodilator activity of (3R)-3-[[[(3-fluorophenyl)[(3,4,5-trifluorophenyl)methyl]amino] carbonyl]oxy]-1-[2-oxo-2-(2-thienyl)ethyl]-1-azoniabicyclo[2.2.2]octane bromide (CHF5407), a potent, long-acting, and selective muscarinic M3 receptor antagonist. J Pharmacol Exp Ther 2010; 335:622-635.

7   Cazzola M, Calzetta L, Matera MG. β_2-adrenoreceptor agonists: current and future direction. Br J Pharmacol 2011; 163:4-17.

8   European Medicines Agency. Summary of product characteristics for Onbrez Breezhaler. Available at: www.ema.europa.eu/docs/en_GB/document_library/EPAR_-_Product_Information/human/001114/WC500053732.pdf. Last accessed October 2012.

9   Arcapta Neohaler [package insert]. East Hanover, NJ: Novartis Pharmaceuticals Corporation; 2011.

10 van Noord JA, Smeets JJ, Drenth BM, et al. 24-hour bronchodilation following a single dose of the novel β_2-agonist olodaterol in COPD. Pulm Pharmacol Ther 2011; 24:666-672.

11 Calverly PM, Anderson JA, Celli B, et al; TORCH investigators. Salmeterol and fluticasone propionate and survival in chronic obstructive pulmonary disease. N Engl J Med 2007; 356:775–789.

12 The Tobacco Use and Dependence Clinical Practice Guideline Panel, Staff, and Consortium Representatives. A clinical practice guideline for treating tobacco use and dependence: A US Public Health Service report. JAMA 2000; 283:3244–3254.

13 Gonzales D, Rennard SI, Nides M, et al; Varenicline Phase 3 Study Group. Varenicline, an alpha4beta2 nicotinic acetylcholine receptor partial agonist, vs sustained-release bupropion and placebo for smoking cessation: a randomized controlled trial. JAMA 2006; 296:47-55.

14 Jorenby DE, Hays JT, Rigotti NA, et al; Varenicline Phase 3 Study Group. Efficacy of varenicline, an alpha4beta2 nicotinic acetylcholine receptor partial agonist, vs placebo or sustained-release bupropion for smoking cessation: a randomized controlled trial. JAMA 2006; 296:56-63.

15 Barnes PJ. Reduced histone deacetylase in COPD: clinical implications. Chest 2006; 129:151–155.

16 Barnes PJ. Theophylline in chronic obstructive pulmonary disease: new horizons. Proc Am Thorac Soc 2005; 2:334–339.

17 Ford PA, Durham A, Russell RE, et al. Treatment effects of low dose theophylline combined with an inhaled corticosteroid in COPD. Chest 2010;137:1338–1344.

18 Cosio BG, Iglesias A, Rios A, et al. Low-dose theophylline enhances the anti-inflammatory effects of steroids during exacerbations of COPD. Thorax 2009; 64:424-429.

19 Barnes PJ, Hansel TT. Prospects for new drugs for chronic obstructive pulmonary disease. Lancet 2004; 364:985–996.

20 Sturton G, Persson C, Barnes PJ. Small airways: an important but neglected target in the treatment of obstructive airway diseases. Trends Pharmacol Sci 2008; 29:340-345.

21 Fan CK. Phosphodiesterase inhibitors in airways disease. Eur J Pharmacol 2006; 533:110–117.

22 Barnes PJ. New therapies for chronic obstructive pulmonary disease. Med Princ Pract 2010; 19:330-338.

23 Barnes PJ. Frontrunners in novel pharmacotherapy of COPD. Curr Opin Pharmacol 2008; 8:300-307.

24 Daliresp [package insert]. St. Louis, MO: Forest Pharmaceuticals, Inc.; 2011.

25 Barnes PJ. Mediators of chronic obstructive pulmonary disease. Pharm Rev 2004; 56:515–548.

26 Leidy NK, Wilcox TK, Jones PW, et al; for the EXACT-PRO Study Group. Development of the EXAcerbations of Chronic Obstructive Pulmonary Disease (EXACT): a Patient Reported Outcome (PRO) measure. Value Health 2010; 13:965-975.

27 Jones RC, Donaldson GC, Chavannes NH, et al. Derivation and validation of a composite index of severity in chronic obstructive pulmonary disease: the DOSE Index. Am J Respir Crit Care Med 2009; 180:1189-1195.

28 Thiberville L, Salaün M, Lachkar S, et al. Human in vivo fluorescence microimaging of the alveolar ducts and sacs during bronchoscopy. Eur Respir J 2009; 33:974-985.

29 van Noord JA, Cornelissen PJ, Aumann JL, et al. The efficacy of tiotropium administered via Respimat Soft Mist Inhaler or HandiHaler in COPD patients. Respir Med 2009; 103:22-29.

30 Asakura Y, Nishimura N, Maezawa K, et al. Effect of switching Tiotropium HandiHaler® to Respimat® Soft Mist™ Inhaler in patients with COPD: the difference of adverse events and usability between inhaler devices. J Aerosol Med Pulm Drug Deliv 2012; epub ahead of print.

31 Rosenberg SR, Kalhan R. An integrated approach to the medical treatment of chronic obstructive pulmonary disease. Med Clin North Am. 2012; 96:811-826.

32 Bach PB, Brown C, Gelfand SE, et al; American College of Physicians–American Society of Internal Medicine; American College of Chest Physicians. Management of acute exacerbations of chronic obstructive pulmonary disease: a summary and appraisal of published evidence. Ann Intern Med 2001; 134:600–620.

33 Ferlay J, Shin H-R, Bray F, et al. Estimates of worldwide burden of cancer in 2008: GLOBOCAN 2008. Int J Cancer 2010; 127:2893-2917.

Printed by Printforce, the Netherlands